E5

Sale

The Complete Question and Answer
Book of Natural Therapy

# The Complete Question and Answer Book of Natural Therapy

BY

GARY NULL and Staff

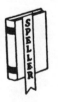

THE HEALTH LIBRARY

ROBERT SPELLER & SONS, PUBLISHERS, INC.
New York, New York 10010

Library of Congress Catalog Card No. 75-187996
ISBN 0-8315-0127-8

First Edition

PRINTED IN THE UNITED STATES OF AMERICA

*To*

*J.I. Rodale and Staff*
*Adelle Davis*
*Carlton Fredericks*
*Gayelord Hauser*
*Linda Clark*
*John Lust*
*Lelord Kordel*
*Carlson Wade*
*Herbert Shelton*
*Paul C. Bragg*
*Bob Hoffman*
*H. E. Kirschner*
*Linus Pauling*
*Ralph Nader*

# TABLE OF CONTENTS

# The Complete Question and Answer
# Book of Natural Therapy

# INTRODUCTION

*The Complete Question and Answer Book of Natural Therapy* is a text that will at once be of valuable service to the layman in search of knowledge pertaining to disease, bodily function and, of course, health and nutrition.

Through this book you, the reader, will be put into immediate contact with information covering everything from the common cold or low back pain to causes and treatments of arthritis and diabetes. From small malady to serious disease, you are offered a look at reasons, theories, facts and fictions that will give you an inside view of what it is to be alive and to desire to live with a healthy body and mind.

To come up with the questions and answers that would tell all in the simplest possible terms was not an easy task. Basically, to cover every area relating to health, nutrition, and natural therapy would be to attempt to fill numbers of overstuffed volumes. The challenge here was to consolidate factual information while, at the same time, bringing together one clear and concise book that would take the reader on a tour of his body, discussing organs from brain to feet and back again and relating how disease affects nutrition and how nutrition affects diease.

*The Complete Question and Answer Book of Natural Therapy* was based on thousands of informal discussions with a cross section of the population in small towns as well as large cities throughout the United States. Everyone from "just plain folks" at the local drug store counter to college professors, nutrition researchers and medical experts were spoken to about common questions that they wanted to ask or that were asked of them most often in regard to health and nhtrition. Age groupings were not a factor, as we interviewed grade school youngsters, teenagers, college students, young businessmen, middle-aged housewives and retired executives. You name the profession or walk of life and we covered it!

1

You will notice certain sections, notably the ones on cancer, heart disease and arthritis, are more detailed than other sections. Also, the format used at times here are questions subdivided into areas with sub-questions. The immense interest and concern relating to cancer, heart disease and arthritis made all this attention and space necessary for these serious diseases.

*The Complete Question and Answer Book of Natural Therapy* is a handbook made up of either exact questions as asked of us, or, when time and space made it necessary, an assimilation of a few questions into one. Look at this as a handbook or if you will as as guide or a treasury. It deserves a valuable place in your library. Use it as a reference book, show it to your friends and give it to your children to take into the classroom. The world of health and nutrition will make just a little more sense after you have digested the important information that this book has to offer.

# HEARING—THE EARS

**Question:** I recently heard a health food store owner tell a gentleman who was having trouble with his hearing to make sure he was getting a necessary vitamin B-complex supply. I had never heard this before. What is the relationship between B-complex and hearing?

**Answer:** Hearing depends on the proper working of a nerve known as the eighth cranial nerve which carries sounds from the inner ear to the brain. Not all forms of deafness are caused by damage to the nerve of hearing. The other parts of the ear apparatus may be involved, too. But for what is known as "nerve deafness" there seems to be no doubt that lack of vitamin B-complex may be a very important cause. For example, we read of cases of beriberi and pellagra, both diseases of vitamin B deficiency—affecting people who do not get in their food enough of the B vitamins. And in both these diseases deafness is one of the symptoms. What happens is that the auditory nerve, which carries sound impressions from the ear to the brain, deteriorates greatly.

Also, we are reminded that no refined sugar can give us one ounce of energy unless thiamin (a B vitamin) is present to break it down from pyruvic acid to energy and carbon dioxide and water. The accumulation of pyruvic acid, for lack of vitamin B, is responsible for ailments including deafness due to nerve disturbance. As well, deposits of cholesterol collecting in the walls of tiny blood vessels may have to do with deafness, especially in persons over middle age. Several of the B vitamins (inositol and choline) are powerful agents against the formation of cholesterol deposits. Lecithin and the unsaturated fatty acids found in vegetable oils also emulsify cholesterol and keep it from depositing where it is not wanted.*

Anyone noticing difficulty hearing what people are saying would be wise to add brewer's yeast in large quantities to his food sup-

---

*Catharyn Ellwood, *Feel Like a Million,* quoted in *Encyclopedia of Common Diseases* by J. I. Rodale and Staff.

plements. Yeast is so rich in all the B vitamins and will aid in preventing nerve deafness.

**Question:** I know that a decline in hearing is accepted as part of growing old by many people. But is there anything specific that I can add to my daily food intake besides the B vitamins that can help me preserve my hearing?

**Answer:** Don't forget the importance of vitamin A. This vitamin affects the ectoderm and the endoderm—those are the parts of the body from which are developed the central nervous system and the mucous membrane. Therefore we can assume with complete authority that vitamin A is of vital importance to the tissues of the inner ear as well as the throat and the chest. Enough vitamin A must be present for the eighth cranial nerve to be healthy.

As we grow old we need more vitamin A and our diets tend to have less of the vitamin in them. The green leafy vegetables and raw fruits may be replaced by cooked vegetables and stewed fruits; the two or more eggs a day may be replaced by refined cereal or toast. Changes like these deprive you of vitamin A and present us with quite a serious problem of vitamin A deficiency. Fish liver oil would be a most healthy addition to your diet as a supplement, as it is rich in vitamin A.

**Question:** I know about vitamin C and its effects on colds. But tell me what, if anything, this vitamin has to do with the protection of my hearing faculties?

**Answer:** Vitamin C is stored in vital organs. This vitamin has something very definite to do with the health of the nerves and of course, this means the nerve of hearing as well as the others. Lack of vitamin C will produce a swelling throughout "Cort's organ" which is in the innermost part of the ear canal. Also tissues of the middle ear store vitamin C and it has been found in treating Ménière's disease—a disorder of the middle ear—that patients in most cases had not been getting nearly enough vitamin C.

**Question:** Please tell me something about the Eustachian tubes and their relation to deafness.

**Answer:** First let us define the Eustachian tubes as the canals in the body which connect the throat with the middle ear. It is their functions to equalize air pressure in the middle ear. When you swallow, the tubes open and allow air to enter and it is for this reason that you experience relief by swallowing during quick changes of altitude. If your Eustachian tubes do not work properly you get the feeling of your ears being stopped up. Your ears are definitely clogged and there is no relief as sounds become dull and distant. You are deaf to a greater or lesser degree.

The deafness problem is related to malformation in size and shape of the Eustachian tubes. The size, contour and tone of a person's Eustachian tubes account for interference with air pressure in the middle ear as well as with blood lymph circulation to different sections of the inner ear. The development of disease in the organ of hearing which resulted in deafness was encouraged by this condition. Now there is a known treatment through an operation which manipulates the size and form to bring the air openings to normal size to allow the air to flow freely and bring sounds into focus loud and clear.

**Question:** I know that tinnitus is the technical name for "ringing in the ears" but not until a family friend was taken with the affliction was I truly aware of its quite present existence. Please tell me more about this malady and its causes.

**Answer:** Tinnitus is a serious ear disorder, rather complicated in kinds and division, and one that causes particular misery of a psychological nature on top of everything else. We say psychological because the sufferer does not necessarily have great pain or a visible wound and therefore does not receive the sympathy he would elicit if exhibiting a broken leg. But, even though it cannot be seen readily, there is a physical basis for most tinnitus.

Sounds such as ringing, buzzing, noise like a waterfall, a jet of steam, a saw, a splash or whistling are present in the ears and can be of such constant degree as to cause extreme desperation. One type of tinnitus is known as "exotic or perotic." This comes from disorders of organs near the auditory apparatus. One of or combinations of arterial and venous disorders have manifestations in the persistent sounds of the inner ear. Another type of tinnitus is called "enotic." Here the sounds are heard by the patient and the sounds are accompanied by deafness, an important factor in diagnosis. Damage to the external ear, such as accumulation of wax or foreign objects is the cause and when removed the symptom disappears. Certain drugs or poisons used in the treatment of disease, quinine for malaria, for example, can cause damage to the internal ear and give rise to tinnitus. And deafness and tinnitus can result from exposure to certain chemicals connected with one's particular occupation. A man working as a gas station attendant is exposed to lead and carbon monoxide frequently; a man employed by a dry cleaning store breathes the toxic benzene fumes frequently.

Another area of tinnitus—"reflex tinnitus"—stems from intriguing avenues. A person can have tinnitus relieved by having his glasses adjusted, a denture refitted or even a tight short collar enlarged.

Finally and most serious is "central tinnitus," wherein the victim hears sounds of all kinds coming from the central auditory canal. They are often violent noises that echo throughout the head and are heard from both ears which further hampers any classification of the cause. Such a condition is often the sign of the development of a serious disorder and should call for a complete neurologic examination.

# SEEING—THE EYES

**Question:** I find that my eyes begin to bother me at the end of a hectic day at the office. I experience blurred vision as well as itching and burning. However, a recent eye examination revealed that I was not in need of glasses. What could be causing my troubles?

**Answer:** A hectic day at the office is most likely producing nervous tension, whether you are conscious of it or not. Nervousness and anxiety stimulate excessive eye muscle activity which in turn gives rise to symptoms of eyestrain. If you are nervously inclined you may be able to overcome these symptoms by simply relaxing. The first step is to plan a relaxing period for each day. Seek quiet, comfortable surroundings, preferably at the same hour in the same place, daily, close your eyes lightly and allow your mind to relax completely. If your eyes sting and itch you can put them at further ease by applying hot compresses. This routine will rest your mind and all body organs as well as your eyes, and it is guaranteed that after a period of time you will be seeing better than ever. Eyestrain, due to tension, a very common thing for working people with pressure jobs will become a thing of the past.

**Question:** I understand that a serious lack of a B vitamin may bring on beriberi. How does that affect the eyes?

**Answer:** It is a serious lack of thiamin (one of the B vitamins) that can cause beriberi. In the eyes, this takes the form of retrobulbar neuritis or what is commonly known as pains behind the eyeball. There may also be many dark spots on the field of vision, probably near the center of this field.

While we are on the subject of B vitamins and eye health, you should know that other vitamins of this group such as riboflavin, niacin, folic acid and pyridoxine are important as well. Without one or all of these essentials in your diet you can experience inflammation of the eyelids, loss of eyelashes, erosion of the eye tissues and clouding of the cornea. When riboflavin is lacking, particularly, the eyelids may itch, eyes grow tired, vision may be poor and

7

cannot be improved by glasses. Also it may be difficult for the individual to see in dim light and there may be extreme sensitivity to light.

**Question:** Does night blindness relate directly to a specific vitamin deficiency?

**Answer:** The lack of vitamin A causes definite eye symptoms and one of these is night blindness. It is known that the normal retina and the choroid (an eye membrane) contain enormous amounts of vitamin A. Apparently, vitamin A is necessary for the process that goes on inside the eye when your body moves from darkness to light, or from light to darkness. So a lack of vitamin A would hinder this process. Night blindness, resulting from vitamin deficiency, may be accompanied by scotomata—that is, dark spots in the field of vision. Also, night blindness is accompanied by dryness of the cornea and the eye tissues, with triangular spots, silver gray and shiny, which are called Bitot's spots, after the physician who first studied them. These conditions are caused by too little vitamin A and can be cured by increasing the amount of vitamin A available for use by the body.

**Question:** I have just learned that my youngest child will need eyeglasses as he is nearsighted. What exactly, in technical terms, is this condition of nearsightedness and what are its causes and cures?

**Answer:** Myopia is the technical term for nearsightedness and it can be defined as a condition in which the individual can see clearly things right beneath his own nose, but cannot see things farther away. The myopic eye is like a camera permanently focused on a close-up. Myopia generally becomes apparent when one is a child or perhaps in the teens. It is caused by an abnormal enlargement of the eye in the diameter from front to rear. This greater length of the diameter of the eye causes the image of what is being seen to be focused in front of the retina rather than on it. As the child grows older this enlargement process gradually ceases.

Many things are blamed for myopia—light used for reading, posture, heredity, diseases and diet deficiencies. The latter seem most responsible as our processed and devitalized modern diets take the important nutrients out of our diet and weaken our physical workings in general. Sufficient quantity of vitamin E is important in preventing myopia. In fact, a high protein diet has correlated with decreased rates of deterioration in eyesight. Along with the pros of a high protein diet, it is important to keep in mind that vitamin E is destroyed in the presence of rancid fats. Potato chips, salt nuts and an assortment of fried foods do nothing to aid healthy eyes. It is to be stressed, in summing up, that if myopia is detected at an early age, the best thing to do would be to begin treatment with vitamin E at once. This nutritional approach to nearsightedness is sound and meaningful.

**Question:** My husband recently had a successful operation for removal of a cataract. In trying to learn more about this disorder I was amazed to find that it afflicts many Americans. Now I want to know where the name—cataract—came from—is there more than one kind and does it cause blindness?

**Answer:** Cataracts have been known down through the ages. The ancient Greeks thought that a cataract was a flow of cloudy fluid in front of the lens. So they named it—waterfall. We have kept the name, even though we know there is no actual flow of water involved. What happens is that the lens of the eye becomes opaque (impenetrable to sight), like a very misty or fogged window glass. The lens is that part of the eye which gathers the rays of light and focuses them on the nerve endings behind it. Apparently what happens in cataract is that cells die or become damaged, turning white. Clusters of these white cells are what you see in the eye with the fully advanced cataract. Cataract is not a "growth." It does not represent cells growing abnormally. It appears to represent cells dying off and becoming useless.

Senile cataract is the most common. The word "senile" is used here because this kind of cataract usually afflicts people who are advanced in age, although, just like gray hair and wrinkles, it can occur in quite young persons as well. Congenital cataract occurs in babies at birth. Diabetic cataract sometimes afflicts diabetics of any age. It is believed to go along with degenerative changes in blood vessels that also occur in diabetics.

Regarding blindness, we say "yes" it does cause it. That does not mean that everyone who gets cataract will become blind. Modern surgery can remove the lens of the eye on which the cataract is spread and replace it with powerful spectacles. But when the cataract is fully developed and not operated on, light cannot pass through and there is no way for the individual to see.

**Question:** I know that all vitamins and good nutrition are important for good eyesight. But in relation to cataract are there any helpful diet hints to nip this condition early and prevent increased difficulty in vision leading to something as radical as surgery?

**Answer:** No one is enthusiastic about surgery. It is believed that cataracts can be prevented by proper diet and care for the eyes. For example, when we find out that the lens containing cataract contains very little or no vitamin C, this seems to indicate something important. One function of vitamin C is to keep repairing the cement between the cells in the lens. It seems likely that lack of C has caused these cells to degenerate and form the cataract. In fact, cataracts in newborn babies are believed to be caused by lack of riboflavin and vitamin C in the mother's own diet. Also, the lack of the mineral, calcium, allows the cataract to form, so that it would be wise to see that you are getting bone meal in your diet, as this is a rich calcium source. And that mineral in the diet seems to be necessary for the expected baby to use his intake of vitamin C correctly.

Another food factor used in treating cataract is chlorophyll. Green plants are more nutritious than dried ones; animals do better on green pasture than dried hay and are healthiest when eating the green grass of summer. The chemical properties of chlorophyll, the green coloring matter of plants, are almost the same as the properties of hemoglobin, the red coloring matter in the blood. The chemical formula differs only in the fact that in the hemoglobin molecule, an atom of iron corresponds to the atom of magnesium in the chlorophyll. In the retardation of cataract the formula of chlorophyll and hemoglobin are so nearly alike. Carotin, a type of chlorophyll, exists in the body of fresh carrots and this, added to diet, fights cataract.

Finally, we have a very large amount of evidence that a diet low in protein is likely to make one susceptible to cataract. Researchers have been able to produce cataracts in animals by feeding them diets in which one or another of the important amino acids (forms of protein) is lacking. The essential amino acids work together—one cannot function without all of them. Adding the missing amino acids to the diet delayed the appearance of the cataracts.

**Question:** If a child is born cross-eyed should a cure be attempted or is it something the child will outgrow naturally?

**Answer:** The condition of crossed eyes or as the medical books call it "strabismus," is a serious one to those afflicted and their families. It is a danger to have the mistaken hope that the child will naturally outgrow this disability. It is much more likely that the condition will worsen to a point where it cannot be corrected. The physical cause of crossed eyes lies in the muscles surrounding the eye. These muscles are equally long and are balanced in equal strength when vision is normal, so that the eye is held in a more or less central position. When one wishes to look to the right or left, or up or down, the muscles contract one side and expand on the other to complete the action. Of course, one who has normal vision is not aware of any effort put forth to accomplish this movement. The adjustment is made subconsciously. In cross-eyed individuals, the muscles are not of equal length or strength. The inner muscle is exerting a force on the eye which the outer muscle cannot match, hence the eye is always looking toward the nose. It is as though the two muscles were engaged in a perpetual tug of war, with the outer muscle always losing.

Briefly, science has come up with four general courses of treatment for crossed eyes. They are: glasses, a patch over the good eye, exercise for the eyes and surgery. The therapy used by a doctor in a case of crossed eyes is aimed at one thing—that is, to equalize the pull of the eye muscles so that the eye in repose is directed straight ahead. The method employed to accomplish this depends upon the severity of the individual condition.

**Question:** I know that glaucoma is the single greatest cause of blindness in the United States. What exactly is this disease and what are its warning symptoms?

**Answer:** Most frightening about glaucoma is that it can cause blindness within a few days. But fortunately if the disease is discovered and treated in time, even acute cases requiring immediate attention can be saved. Glaucoma is increased pressure inside the eye and may lead to serious loss of vision without the person even suspecting anything is wrong. The eye has its own built-in mechanism which secretes a watery fluid called "aqueous." This "aqueous" is important to the nourishment of the eyes. Just as there is a secretion mechanism within the eyes, so also is there a drainage channel to allow a steady flow of the "aqueous" out of the eye. If this drainage channel is inadequate or gets plugged up for some reason, the fluid collecting within the eye can't get out readily enough and the pressure inside the eye gets higher and higher. When the fluid pressure inside the eye becomes greater there is more strain on the wall of the eyeball. Especially vulnerable is the optic nerve which is located on the back wall of the eyeball. Increased pressure on the optic nerve causes damage to the optic nerve fibers; as a result of this damage, the person's vision slowly decreases. The loss of vision may be so gradual that the person himself isn't conscious of it until a great deal of damage has occurred.

Sometimes there are warning symptoms of early glaucoma and these should not be ignored. Attacks of blurred vision, which may or may not be accompanied by redness of the eyes, pains, rainbow halos around lights at night, headaches, vertigo or nausea, as well as early morning pains in the eyes, should be examined. Also, the inability to adjust to darkened rooms and loss of peripheral vision —that is, vision at the sides—when the range of vision has become so narrowed that one can see only the object at which he is directly looking, these are both causes worth looking into. And finally, difficulty with vision which makes one try frequent changes of glasses, none of which are comfortable.

Glaucoma is still basically a disease with the usual absence of warning signs until the condition has progressed to the point where vision is affected. Therefore we can say that any increased pressure in the eyes should be checked into.

**Question:** Can you give me a concise idea of what constitutes a satisfactory diet so that I may take care of my eyes properly, from day to day?

**Answer:** Here's where vitamin C pops right up to the very forefront, to begin with. Vitamin C is important for good health. For one, cataract can be prevented by the proper intake and maintenance of vitamin C. And if scurvy sets in as a result of vitamin C deficiency there are hemorrhages of the eyelids and eye tissues. The eyes have a tendency to water, the conjunctival membranes grow dry and there may be a softening or ulceration of the cornea. Also, we know that there are large amounts of vitamin C in the lens and other parts of the normal eye. Vitamin D is important and if you live in the north, particularly supplement your diet with fish liver oils, as the D vitamin is the one our body manufactures from the ultra-violet rays of the sun. If there is no sunshine all year round, you need D supplements.

Eat whole grain cereals, lots of liver or kidney and supplement your diet with desiccated liver or brewer's yeast for those extra B vitamins. Parsley, endive, watercress, raw spinach, lots of fresh fruit—all of these will see that you get the necessary vitamins to aid you in keeping your eye health.

### BIBLIOGRAPHY

Bates, M. D., W. H., *Better Eyesight Without Glasses,* Pyramid Books.

Bourne, Geoffrey, *Biochemistry and Physiology of Nutrition,* Academic Press.

Clark, Linda, *Get Well Naturally,* Arc Books, Inc.

Flatto, Edwin, *The Restoration of Health—Nature's Way,* Pyramid Books.

Poynter, C. W. M., *Congenital Anomalies of the Arteries and Veins of the Human Body,* University of Nebraska Press.

Rodale, J. I. and staff, *The Encyclopedia of Common Diseases,* Rodale Books, Inc.

# HAIR AND BALDNESS

**Question:** Although there are cases of women losing their hair, I understand that baldness is basically a problem that usually confines itself to men. Can you give me some possible reasons for this phenomenon?

**Answer:** This is an interesting question. For years specialists have bandied about theories of baldness being more predominant in men than in women and they have come up with no definite answers. And for each case studied and each cause explored and established there can be found examples counteracting what has been learned. In any case, it seems very right to say that baldness is a natural phenomenon, which, unless a method is found to prevent it, is bound to occur in many a male.

We can look at some theories. Some say it is purely hereditary, passed down from man to man, something left over from man's early ancestry. Others talk of the male sex hormones, which stimulate oil-producing glands in the skin, changing the amount or quality of the oil they produce, and thus contributing to baldness. And then there is the matter of circulation, which is regrowth being stimulated through massage, frequent brushing and methods of bringing the blood into the hair region. It is believed that this "exercise" of the hair is practiced by woman much more. From earliest childhood, the woman has been exercising her hair, while men's hair needs no such tending for appearances' sake. The reason men do not lose their hair on the sides and in the back is that these regions receive friction from the pillow at night, while the crown does not. Finally, there are seemingly irrelevant speculations as to why men become bald while women do not. Perhaps it is the tight collars men wear, while women as a rule do not. Or could it be the fact that women, in general, have wider arteries then men? We have heard this is so, and this results in better circulation among women.

All told, in regard to the sexes, a careless diet, whether male or female, can be accepted as the very basic cause of all baldness.

Somehow the person who is a victim of baldness is short of some food element which is a vital part of the body's hair-growing formula.

**Question:** What do scalp muscles have to do with baldness?

**Answer:** Having developed scalp muscles can only help in preventing baldness. Scalps that receive exercise develop muscles and these muscles under the scalp have a rich supply of blood vessels which bring additional blood needed by the hair follicles for healthy hair. Lots of thriving blood vessels under the scalp mean only good things for the hair. The massage therapy is often recommended for a good head of hair or certainly as a stimulant for falling hair. A special massage is fine, but "exercise", to keep those scalp muscles with its blood vessels happy, should be practiced every day. Simply try to move your scalp consciously by wrinkling your forehead and attempting to move your ears. Do this each morning and evening for a few minutes. It doesn't cost anything and scientific evidence says it should help you retain your hair.

**Question:** Is there any particular vitamin that is especially kind to the hair?

**Answer:** The use of the B vitamin, inositol, in combination with other sources of B vitamins is recommended in treating baldness. In almost every case in which inositol therapy was administered, the patient reported that the hair took on a new freshness and stopped falling out. In some cases new hair growth was obvious within a month. Recommended for baldness prevention was a teaspoon of inositol daily, added to a quart of fortified milk. It was thought the other vitamins and protein in this fortified milk would have something to do with the hair growth as well as the inositol. But the basic mystery of baldness pops up here as one man in a group of 48 sports enormous amounts of hair, while some men did not grow a single wisp.*

We know that the B vitamins are vital to bodily health, especially for nerves and internal organs. Extra intake of B vitamins in the form of brewer's yeast, wheat germ, kidney and liver, can only bring added good health. Try inositol as a weapon against

---

*Adelle Davis, *Let's Eat Right To Keep Fit.*

hair loss and make sure your diet is always rich in all B vitamins.
Even if you are not bothered by falling hair now, the B group
can serve as a preventive measure.

**Question:** What is the feeling about tonics and lotions in relation to proper hair health and to baldness as well?

**Answer:** It is the opinion of most experts that there is nothing
you can rub on your head, paint on your head or spray on your
head that will bring back lost hair. If you do insist on treating
your baldness from the outside, you might as well settle for a
toupee or hairpiece, because it's the only way you'll ever cover
your scalp with hair. If you are willing to try nutrition, you might
be successful in growing new hair or halting the mass desertion of
hair, by reducing your salt intake. Sodium chloride (salt) in excess in a diet can cause the clogging up of the scalp tissues, thus
preventing their function of growing hair. Try inositol, exercising
of scalp muscles—anything but using worthless, sometimes harmful tonics, lotions and cosmetic preparations. You should know
your hair intimately. If it is extremely sensitive and there is chance
of hair loss occurring, even soaps and shampoos can be harmful
as they tend to alkalize a normally acid scalp and destroy the
natural oils. There are many chemicals used that may cause
trouble—the oils in bay rum, the synthetic perfumes in brilliantine,
the various oils and resins in creams and wave preparations. Also
shampoos contain perfume and various sulphur mixtures. Cocoa-
nut oil shampoos, for one, are perfumed with several synthetic
oils, any one of which may be harmful to individual users. And
hair dyes, rinses and permanent wave lotions, all ploys of the hair-
dresser's trade, are not assets to women's hair conditioning.

If hair is allowed to grow unmolested by any solution or process, letting the natural oils do the work, along with frequent brushing and exercising of the scalp, it will keep its natural luster. Combine this with a well balanced diet, rich in the essential vitamins
and minerals and your hair as well as your entire body will benefit. The hair, like the rest of our body must be fed, and it responds best to those elements of food which are natural and vital
to its life and health.

## BIBLIOGRAPHY

Goodman, Herman, *Your Hair: Its Health, Beauty and Growth*, Emerson Books.

Hiller, Norman G., *The Life and Beauty of Your Hair*, Devin-Adair Co.

Lubowe, Irwin Irville, *New Hope for Your Hair*, Dutton Press.

Nessler, Charles, *The Story of Hair: Its Purpose and Preservation*, Boni and Liveright Pub.

Parrotto, Anthony J., *Baldness, Grayness and Dandruff*, Whitmore Pub.

Piowonka, James M., *You Can Help Yourself to Beauty*, Health Research Pub.

Weinberg, Harriet, *The Science of Hair Culture*, Universal Pub.

# TEETH AND DECAY

**Question:** What is actually known about the causes of tooth decay?

**Answer:** The large amount of refined foods eaten today contain large amounts of carbohydrates (sugar and starches). When being eaten these foods leave particles in the mouth and these particles become entrapped on the surface of the teeth.

To further understand this, let's take a look at a controlled diet and its effect on tooth decay. A group of children between the ages of 4 and 9 live in the institution, Hopewood House. They have been there since the earliest months of life. Their surroundings are healthful. They live as much as possible as if they were in their own homes, rather than an institution. The home is located on a 750-acre estate in the southern highlands of New South Wales, Australia. The diet the children eat consists of: wholemeal bread, wholemeal biscuits, wholemeal porridge, wheat germ, fruits, fresh and dried vegetables (cooked and raw), a small amount of meat, butter, eggs, cheese, milk and fruit juices. Every child takes vitamins and is allowed a little honey or molasses and occasionally, nuts. Food is taken as much as possible in its natural state and notable for their absence from the diet were white and brown sugar, white flour products, including cake and biscuits and any combination of these items. No tea was used. The water was drawn from the town supply and there appeared to be no fluoride in it. Tests and examinations were made of all the children for a period of about five years. It was found that of 81 children, 63 had no tooth decay. This proportion of children without decay is far in excess of those in other groups throughout Australia, Canada and New Zealand. The teeth of the group as a whole were remarkable for the small number of decay spots. No child had more than 6 teeth needing care. The rates of decay beginning and proceeding in the mouths of these children were very far below those of the population, in general. The outstanding difference in comparison was

18

the nature of the diet. The absence of foods containing carbohydrates proved to foster healthy teeth.*

Also, whatever the diet, it is most important to visit your dentist regularly and be aware of the proper way to brush your teeth and the best type of toothbrush to use to fit your needs. Just as every person is very different, so are their mouths and the teeth within them.

**Question:** Are the B vitamins more than just a common part of the necessary diet that will curtail tooth decay and stimulate healthy teeth?

**Answer:** Yes, particularly the vitamin known as B6 (pyridoxine). In relation to teeth care, this specific vitamin is known to be able to maintain a climate of bacterial flora which is beneficial to the proper development and good health of the teeth. This climate of bacterial flora, known as lactobacilli most specifically, which would need vitamin B6 as an essential nutrient, was multiplying rapidly with the extra B6 dosage. Its growth works to ease out and eliminate certain bacteria which are detrimental to the health of the teeth. In pregnant women there is a large amount of cortisone secreted from the adrenals. The cortisone interferes with the body's ability to use vitamin B6. And the cortisone administered to hospitalized children was interfering with the availability of the vitamin B6 to the tissues and aiding in tooth decay. Therefore, in whatever circumstances cortisone in one's body would be on the increase, and addition of B6 to the diet would be reasonable. Sugarcane is particularly high in B6 as is the molasses prepared from sugarcane.

**Question:** How important is fluoride in water supply in relation to the maintenance of healthy teeth?

**Answer:** The prevention of decay by the use of fluorides in the drinking water or by even painting them on the teeth can be cheap and simple—but that's of importance only when it's effective which is not at all very often and certainly not for everyone. While fluoridation of water may well reduce or delay dental decay in

---

*Medical Journal of Australia as quoted in *Encyclopedia of Common Diseases* by J. I. Rodale and Staff.

very young children, its effects on the health of older people, infants and ill people have not been studied sufficiently to warrant taking a chance on artificial fluoridation.

Experiments with rats have shown them remaining as healthy or not and with or without good teeth in no direct relation to an intake of fluoride. And in 1962, our Public Health Department reported that the children in Newburgh, New York, where water was first fluoridated, had slightly more decay after fluoridation than before. In Baltimore, Maryland, where water had been fluoridated since 1952, rampant decay has steadily increased. In Puerto Rico, not only has tooth decay increased since fluoridation of the water supply, but 64 percent of adolescent boys have mottled, permanently stained teeth from fluoride excess, the ugly brown spots ruining every smile. Fluorine has been shown to be harmful to many of the body's enzyme systems; and drinking fluoridated water has become a common cause of allergies. It increases the brittleness of teeth and bones. There is some indication it may damage the chromosomes. When water is fluoridated, some of the fluorine combines with magnesium to form magnesium fluoride, an insoluble salt which cannot be absorbed by the intestine. This can produce a deficiency of magnesium, and it is known that potassium leaves the cells when magnesium is deficient. Thus it is not surprising to learn that deaths from heart disease have increased in areas where the water is fluoridated. Certainly the choice as to whether fluorine is to be included in the diet should be left to each individual and not be imposed upon him by having the entire water supply fluoridated at great cost to the taxpayer.*

**Question:** I know that orthodontics is a flourishing branch of dentistry today and that this specialization is good for children or adults when their teeth are in trouble. But when does one know that it's time to make the move from friendly family dentist to orthodontic doctor?

**Answer:** Orthodontics is devoted to the prevention and correction of malocclusion of the teeth and other associated abnormalities and deformities. Malocclusion is defined in the medical dictionary as "occlusion of teeth in positions not comfortable to ana-

---

*Adelle Davis, *Let's Eat Right To Keep Fit.*

tomical rule." This means that if your teeth do not meet in such a way as to give you a fully functioning "bite" as well as good appearance, you have malocclusion. When your "bite" is ineffective, when your teeth are growing so far out of line with one another and with the plane in which they function that you cannot use your teeth as you should—that is also malocclusion.

Children are the people most often going to orthodontists, so you should be aware of some of the causes of malocclusion in youngsters. If abnormality is indicated by all means take them to a trained expert. First, pay close attention to baby teeth. If any are lost prematurely, take the child to an orthodontist as he will be able to supply you with a "space maintainer" which will provide and maintain room for later teeth. Second, prolonged retention of baby teeth can only prevent the permanent teeth from coming into place as they are deflected out of their proper course. Third, pay close attention to the loss of a permanent tooth before the entire set of permanent teeth has grown in, for here again the space will tend to close rapidly, throwing out of line the teeth in that side of the jaw which are still coming through the gums. Also be on the lookout for extra teeth that fail to come in altogether. This can also result in malocclusion.

**Question:** What relation—if any—does nutrition have to malocclusion?

**Answer:** While it is believed that heredity, primarily in regard to facial structure, can have its direct relation to malocclusion, there are certainly environmental factors that are most important. The serving of a consistently bad diet can cause degeneration of the bony structure quickly in children, resulting in something more serious than tooth decay—the need for orthodontic treatment. The ideal solution would be for mother and father to be eating a primitive diet, one free of refined foods, and to pass this diet on to their children and their children's children. But realistically in America today, you cannot eat a primitive diet. The very seeds you put in your garden bear the mark of civilization on them. But you can plan your meals so that a very minimum of processed food appears on your table. You can learn how to preserve most food value by cooking methods and you can serve quantities of raw food. A strong, functioning bone structure and good teeth go hand in hand with natural, unrefined foods.

**Question:** My young son goes to grade school and is beginning to have decay problems. I know he eats a lot of candy at snack time.How do you prevent this, without tempting the fates, and making him want the candy even more and taking it, while you have little or no control over this part of his diet?

**Answer:** A good question and one which can be answered by using a bit of psychology. It would be advisable to go to the next PTA meeting, or even better to arrange a personal meeting with your child's teacher. Suggest that they create something in the classroom such as "health snack time," a kind of happening that would exclude candy and any mention of sweets, of course. Each day one child would bring a treat for the entire class and serve it himself. These treats could consist of carrot or celery strips, apple or orange wedges, dried prunes, raisins, dried apricots, peaches or fresh fruits in season. Setting up this kind of community food-fest, all with the most nutritious ingredients, will start a new routine at a young age, and the children will be less and less apt to bring sweets to school for a snack. They won't ask you for the candy as often and they won't think of buying it at the local store and sneaking it to school. They will be prone to accepting the idea of good nutrition readily.

# THE GUMS

**Question:** I know that people who are past middle age are faced with the prospect of losing all their teeth as a result of unhealthy gums and not because of tooth decay exclusively. What are the basic causes that contribute to gum deterioration?

**Answer:** First, gum trouble—known as periodontal disease, can be directly related to how one's teeth perform their functions of biting and chewing. Teeth that are too big or too small for their supporting gum structure, teeth that do not meet properly in a "bite" so that much of the force of the bite is lost, teeth that are clenched or ground because of nervous habits are likely to be responsible for much of gum trouble. Also, irritants on the inside of the mouth stemming from impaction of food, tartar on the teeth, and mechanical irritants, such as dentures that don't fit and rub against the gums, chemical irritants, improper mouth breathing, improper tooth brushing—all these help to bring on trouble with gums.

Then too there are problems having to do solely with body health. Faulty nutrition may mean that the body is too acid or too alkaline; that there is vitamin or mineral deficiency or both; chronic diseases, gland disorders, anemias, allergies or sensitivity to drugs; pregnancy and psychological causes. Vitamin C is the single most important food factor for gum health, vitamin A and vitamin B being almost as important, as well as calcium and the other minerals that are necessary for bone health. Much of our trouble with gums arises from the fact that jawbones disintegrate and wear away so that the whole mouth and tooth structure is thrown out of alignment. American diets are notoriously short on calcium, so necessary for healthy bone structure.

**Question:** Please tell me some more about bleeding gums. I know that when I brush my teeth in the morning I will occasionally draw blood, but I never really give it much thought.

**Answer:** You should see your dentist about bleeding gums and if necessary see a specialist, a periodontist. Bleeding gums

23

indicate a lack of proper nutriments so necessary to a healthy mouth. Most specifically, bleeding gums seem to show an almost immediate and positive response to the addition of vitamin C. Lack of C will be exhibited by puffy and spongy gums and can result in dead cells in the gum tissue—cells that ever-present bacteria live off. But treatment and dosage with C should be followed with a physician's guidance. Also protein deficiency results in increased incidence of periodontal disease. This is due to reduced resistance to infection and impaired healing. If you remember that protein actually supplies the raw materials for building tissue in the same way that bricks provide the raw material for building a wall, its importance in maintaining healthy gums becomes clear. And once again, whether it be a problem of sore or bleeding gums or let's say, colitis, the cure still lies in a program of complete nutrition, not just one vitamin for a few weeks, but all of the vitamins all of the time—either in the foods we eat or natural supplements.

**Question:** What is the difference between gingivitis and pyorrhea and tell me some more about what is happening when these gum disorders are functioning?

**Answer:** Gingivitis is the technical term for inflammation of the gums whereas pyorrhea is the term for the more serious gum disorders. It can be defined as chronic gingivitis. In pyorrhea the gums become swollen and red, they bleed easily and are tender to the touch. As the disease progresses, the gum tissues detach themselves gradually from the teeth, the gums become thick, hard and leathery and eventually the bony foundation of the tooth roots is destroyed, the teeth become loose and must be extracted. The disease resembles tuberculosis in that it progresses very slowly, giving no warning by pain or discomfort. Pyorrhea can be detected though, as early as five years before it becomes serious, by the use of X-ray. Tooth decay is a disease of youth, claiming the majority of its victims as teenagers; gingivitis affects young and old, but it is pyorrhea that is most specifically a disease of middle age and old age, which leads one to believe that it is a degenerative disease and hence can be prevented.

**Question:** What causes pyorrhea and what can help prevent it?

**Answer:** This is important to know, for as you would probably be surprised to learn, more teeth are lost because of pyorrhea than because of tooth decay. And very often pyorrhea is not at all accompanied by tooth decay. There are mechanical reasons for some cases. Chewing always on one side of the mouth can bring it on. Malocclusion can produce pyorrhea, because the stresses and strains of chewing can work havoc with teeth and gums alike when the teeth are not arranged in the proper pattern to share these stresses. Excessive tartar can cause pyorrhea by accumulating along the gums and irritating them until pus pockets are formed. Yet we are acquainted with people who take meticulous care of their mouth, brushing the teeth very carefully after each meal and these folks still have excessive tartar on their teeth which makes them candidates for pyorrhea as well. Vincent's disease or trench mouth results in ulcers of the gums,, mouth and throat, which are extremely painful and pus-laden, taking weeks or even months to totally cure.

Look to your vitamins and minerals. A proper amount helps prevent pyorrhea while a lack of essentials over a period of time promotes the disease. Vitamin A affects the nerves in the body and it is possible that pyorrhea could start when the relationship between nerves and nutrition in the mouth becomes weak because of the A deficiency. Also, vitamin A should be present liberally in the diet of expectant mothers and milk-secreting mothers and of their offspring, at least up to puberty, in order to insure that the gum epithelium and alveolar bone are properly formed. People afflicted with pellagra—a vitamin B deficiency disease—displayed a high percentage of Vincent's disease. And once given niacin (a B vitamin), almost all redness and soreness disappeared immediately. Vitamin C is most essential in fighting pyorrhea because of the serious gum disease that accompanies scurvy. A culture whose diet is lacking in large quantities of fresh fruits and vegetables would tend towards pyorrhea because of the great vitamin C deficiency. Vitamin C deficiency destroys the body's ability to rebuild tissues and fibers such as those of the gums.

Regarding mineral content, a calcium-phosphorus balance is an important consideration. A high phosphorus-low calcium ratio seems to be present in pyorrhea patients. That is, the diets contained far too much phosphorus in relation to the amount of cal-

cium. The high phosphorus pulls the calcium out of the body
with loss of bone density. Therefore sources of calcium—milk and
green leafy vegetables, should be ever present in the diet in balanced relation to meat and cereal intake. This is necessary in
preventing pyorrhea and can only aid bodily health.

No one wants to lose teeth and have his gums destroyed, so that
pyorrhea is a major concern to anyone growing older. And to combat it is to have a balanced intake of the most important vitamins.
Vitamins A and D are contained in fish liver oil. All the B vitamins
are in brewer's yeast and desiccated liver. Vitamin C is most
abundant in rose hips and other natural C supplements. The
proper ratio of calcium and phosphorus is found in bone meal,
along with other important minerals. You can't get along without
all of them. And by taking just one or two of these supplements, you may be leaving out the very vitamin or mineral in which
you are deficient. So consult with your physician. If it is all planned
when the teeth are relatively healthy and the gums firm and pink,
gingivitis or the more serious pyorrhea will be no problem at all.
Only neglect will encourage these diseases to fester in the mouth.

BIBLIOGRAPHY

Allport, Walter Webb, *Diseases of the Teeth,* Barnet and Clarke
Pub.

Charney, Margaret Stella, *Nutrition,* Houghton Mifflin Co.

Clark, Linda, *Get Well Naturally,* Arc Books, Inc.

Davis, Adelle, *Let's Eat Right to Keep Fit,* Signet Books.

Dunning, James Morse, *Principles of Dental Health,* Harvard University Press.

Hawkins, Harold Fuller, *Applied Nutrition,* California Institute
Press.

MacLeod, Florence Louise, *Fat-Soluble Vitamin and Calcium in
Nutrition,* Columbia University Thesis.

Price, Weston, *Nutrition and Physical Degeneration,* The Lee
Foundation for Nutritional Research.

Warmbrand, Max, *The Encyclopedia of Natural Health,* Groton
Press.

# THE FEET

**Question:** Is it true that the way we stand and walk has a lot to do with the health of our feet?

**Answer:** The way we walk and stand has more to do with the health of our feet than any other one factor. The weight of your body should be borne on the outside arch of the foot which is made of bone for the express purpose of bearing weight. The inside arch is made mostly of ligaments and muscles. When we walk incorrectly and stand with an incorrect posture, the weight is thrown instead on the inside arch. Muscles and ligaments endure all they can, and then give way, resulting in fallen arches which is one of the most painful conditions known and may involve all types of dreadful apparatus necessary to bring relief. The purpose of these contraptions is, of course, to take the place of the muscles that have collapsed. Exercise is important, too, in curing fallen arches, as well as specially designed shoes. All of them are very expensive and painful.

To prevent foot trouble, preventive measures should begin in early childhood. And this brings attention to posture, which is most important. One's feet should at all times be straight—that is, parallel to one another, rather than turned out or turned in. Pigeon-toes suggest immediately that something is wrong and the pigeon-toed child should be taken to the doctor. When the toes turn out in walking or standing, the weight of the body is thrown on the inner arch which sooner or later is bound to give way. So the first and most important exercise for healthy feet is learning to walk and stand with feet parallel. When we take a step the weight should be first on the heel, then as we go forward, it is transferred to the outer arch and finally to the great toe.

It is impossible to walk correctly unless you have comfortable shoes. Women should realize that technically it is impossible for one to walk comfortably in high heels. Regardless of whether you are holding your feet correctly parallel, they must slip forward in your shoes due to the height of the heel. And many of the foot troubles of modern women are concentrated in the forepart of the foot which is that part which is twisted and deformed by high heels. There is considerable controversy regarding what constitutes correct shoes. They should be big enough and right here is where so many foot troubles have their start in childhood when little feet are growing rapidly, getting too big for shoes, long before the shoes wear out. Some shoe salesmen would recommend a shoe with a little more width, some with more length and others with a compactness instead of a roominess. Everyone has different ideas in relation to the individual's size and shape of feet. But one thing is certain, if we are going to stand and walk comfortably the materials housing our feet must be totally comfortable and supportive.

**Question:** How will I know when my children of grade school age definitely need a new pair of shoes?

**Answer:** Children's shoes should be replaced as soon as there is the slightest indication that they are too small. The fitting should be carefully made, with the child standing, so that the full weight is on the feet. There should be the width of an adult's thumb between the toes and the end of the shoe. And since you never know how fast your child is growing during any given time, you should make frequent examinations between shopping trips, just to make sure that junior's feet still have enough room inside his shoes. In general, it appears that shoes should be firm enough to give support, yet should not be made of stiff unyielding leather which may be appealing because of its durability. Nor should sneakers be worn a great deal of the time. If your child finds that sneakers are comfortable during the summer, make sure that he wears leather shoes part of the time, for sneakers, or tennis shoes, do not give enough support for constant wear. Until the age of 16, children's shoes should be renewed every 3 or 4 months, if you want to be certain their shoes are not too small. Hand-me-downs are not advised when it comes to shoes. No one, child or adult, should wear shoes that someone else has been wearing. Heels should be straightened whenever they seem to be run over. And, incidentally, heels worn down either on the outside or the inside are an indication that posture is poor and feet are not functioning as they should.

The first evidence of badly fitted shoes appears on the skin.

Redness or blisters anywhere on the foot indicate friction or pressure which means poor fit. Even in children, corns and calluses will develop, indicating that the foot-gear is possibly causing friction or pressure at one particular point and that the shoes that cause trouble should be thrown away. If the child is regularly getting the proper shoes and still has complaints about his feet not feeling comfortable, it may be something that would require the care of a physician and not a shoe salesman. Foot trouble, especially in children, should not be neglected for an instant.

**Question:** I work in a department store and am either standing behind a counter or moving between floors all day long. What are some basic rules of health to protect my feet from harm?

**Answer:** To begin with, select shoes and hose that fit properly. Tight shoes cause pressure usually and shoes that are too large cause friction. The heels of shoes should be kept straight. Your shoes should be well supported through the arch of the foot. If not feet will tend to flatten when you stand up. When standing, as you do, for long periods, place the feet 2 to 4 inches apart, point them straight ahead and support the weight on the outside of the feet. When walking, keep the feet parallel and pointed straight ahead. In stepping forward, the weight should fall on the heel first, whereupon the body is carried forward over the foot, weight being applied along the outside of the foot from the heel to the small toe and finally across the forward part of the great toe. Fallen arches are the result of weakened leg muscles which allow the main or lengthwise arch in the foot to sag. An orthopedic surgeon should be consulted about this condition, if it affects you, as special treatment is needed. When you are bathing proper attention is most important to foot care. The feet should be washed with warm water and then thoroughly dried. The toenails should be cut straight across and not too short. Also, you should give immediate attention to all wounds and blisters in order to prevent serious consequences. And even though you've been on your feet all day, some proper exercise at home is quite good. Try strengthening the arches by bending the toes—best accomplished by picking up small objects such as marbles, with the toes.

**Question:** What exactly is the condition popularly known as Athlete's Foot?

**Answer:** Athlete's foot, also known as ringworm, is a skin disease caused by fungus. Fungus thrives best in a warm, moist, dark environment, just the kind the inside of a shoe provides. The raising of the skin's resistance by using food supplements rich in vitamins C and A is one of the means of avoiding this problem. Another is frequent soaking of the feet, and fresh, clean socks or stockings daily so that the feet will stay dry in the shoes. This measure is also most effective in eliminating offensive foot odors.

**Question:** I live year round in a fairly warm climate near the beach. My footwear is generally casual and I have been using the thong-type sandal, instead of shoes, regularly. Will they do my feet any harm over a period of time?

**Answer:** A good question, because in today's society the bent towards casualness, away from formality, has even reflected itself in what people are wearing on their feet. The thong-type sandal was extensively worn by the ancient Greeks and Romans, and it is still widely used throughout Central and South America and in the Far East, not to exclude the United States. The thong sandal when it is properly made is truly non-deforming foot-gear. The thong between the great and second toe permits the toes perfect freedom and expansibility. In recent years thong-type sandals have become popular as beach wear. But, if leather is used the usual sole leather is not satisfactory, for, unless leather permits flexibility throughout the foot, the musculature soon suffers. Flexible belt leather should be used for the sole. Thong-type sandals are easily made. A single layer of belt sole leather should be cut out to an outline of the bare foot increased on all sides by a quarter of an inch. With a chisel two slits, three-sixteenths of an inch apart, are cut in the sole space between the great and second toe. Slits are cut on the edge of the sole on either side of the foot, behind the great and little toe joints respectively. Two other slits are cut on the edge of the sole in front of the ankle bones. Strap leather thongs are then woven through the slits and the foot is firmly bound to the sole. Homemade sandals can be effective. It is the factory output, mass-produced sandal that will cause harm.

BIBLIOGRAPHY

Bourne, Aleck William, *Health of the Future*, Penguin Books.

Carelton, Frank J., *Shoes and Feet*, York, Pa. Press of Printing.

LaLanne, Jack, *The Jack LaLanne Way to Vibrant Good Health*, Arc Books, Inc.

Morton, Dudley Joy, *The Human Foot— Its Evolution, Physiology and Function Disorders*, Columbia University Press.

Murray, Alan E., *Shoes and Feet to Boot*, Chapel Hill Pub.

Rossi, William A., *Podometrics: A New Approach to Shoes and Feet*, Hide and Leather Pub. Co.

Scholl, William Mathias, *Dictionary of the Feet,* Foot Specialist Pub. Co.

# THE SKIN

**Question:** What can begin to cause skin irritations of an every-day nature? I ask this because I am a 30 year old housewife that has frequent sores on the skin, seemingly caused by my daily household activities.

**Answer:** Consider the skin disorder known as contact dermatitis or more simply, skin disease resulting from the touch of an object. This can explain soreness if one is talking about disorder associated with everyday household objects and activities. Dermatitis conditions can be difficult and a look at this problem is a good place to begin. The dialing of a telephone resulting in a ring of blisters around the index finger; the turning of a car key; and the zipping of a brief case causing itchy blisters that are bothersome. These are indicative of contact dermatitis. A doctor investigating the disorder must puzzle out, from just where the sores appear and how they develop, what object one would contact only in these spots and whether it is liquid or solid, round or flat, rod or rope etc. Then, to cooperate, the patient must try to record his every contact throughout the day, he must remember any changes that might have occurred in his daily schedule—any clue he can offer might carry in it the key to his problem. Imagine, of the thousands of things one touches in a day, narrowing the suspects down to the dial of a telephone! All age groups are subject to contact dermatitis. Even infants of a few weeks of age have been known to be sensitive to their mothers' lipstick. Incidence has shown dermatitis to be more prevalent in later life than in early years. Also, women are known to be more susceptible than men—the percentage of women who suffer from contact dermatitis is almost double that of men. Though it has not been proven, it is supposed that the large variety of cosmetics, hair dyes and perfumes employed by women account for this difference. The materials which are most likely to penetrate the skin are usually oily in character—plant oils or certain lubricating oils cling to the fatty covering of the skin and dissolve more readily than water soluble materials. Certain dyes have the ability to become fixed in the horny layer of the skin. During their prolonged stay the elements of the dyes come into intimate contact with the sensitive cells, and eruption of tiny blisters often results. Other common offenders are metallic salt and local anesthetics. All of these sources are easily contacted in an ordinary day's activities. The plants which give off oils which cause dermatitis are common enough: live oak, sumac, chrysanthemums, ragweed, certain blubs, etc. The dyes are everywhere: leather shoes, wallets, belts, colored clothing, furs, gloves and many more objects that are dyed including soaps, fingernail polishes, hair rinses, toilet tissues, powders and lipsticks. Among the metals, nickel and aluminum are the worst offenders. It seems unlikely that one would go through a typical day at home without at least coming into contact with some of the above mentioned. It's when that unexplained irritation pops up that all possible causes must be investigated. And the realistic possibility of contact dermatitis must be examined.

**Question:** Can one really get clean without the use of soap?

**Answer:** There are many critics of commercial soap use and they have solid grounds to illustrate their dissatisfactions. It is well known that soap can cause dermatitis in sensitive persons and in those not so sensitive, who are frequently exposed. The use of soap is likely to aggravate any existing skin problem no matter what its original cause. Sensitivity to soap is usually attributed to coloring matter, or the medications and perfumes included in various kinds. But the basic composition of soap makes it a natural troublemaker. The soap molecule includes an oil soluble fatty acid and a water soluble alkali. The alkali softens and dissolves the protective layers of the skin, and both it and the fatty acid are likely to produce skin irritation. Since we know that soap isn't essential in cleansing the body it would be foolish to invite the problems of soap dermatitis by using it.

**Question:** I watch television and read magazines with detergent advertisements proclaiming "be kind to your hands" all over the place. Is this true or simply a ploy of advertising agencies in order to sell the products?

**Answer:** The most powerful claim a detergent can make, even more important than whether or not it is an effective cleaner, is that it is kinder to hands. Along with the advertised quick efficiency of modern detergents has come the almost universal complaint that they literally eat into the skin. One of the most common points of attack is the tender part under the fingernails. Severe hemorrhages and great pain under the fingernails have resulted from the irritant factor in detergents. And this happened in cases where rubber gloves were known to be used while washing the dishes. It is suggested that one wear cotton gloves under rubber gloves when exposing the hands to detergent water. Contact with detergent solutions damages keratin, a fibrous protein that forms the outer coating of the skin. When the harsh chemicals contained in detergents eat away this protective substance, the tender underlayers of the skin are defenseless against a similar attack. Detergents can cause serious hand dermatitis with some detergent users more susceptible to trouble than others. For example, they are more likely to irritate the skin of blondes than brunettes; men are more susceptible to irritation than females; Negroes are least susceptible. The condition of the skin is important; oily skins are less easily affected than dry skins, and excess perspiration increases chances of contacting dermatitis and makes existing hand dermatitis worse.

If one is exposed to detergent solutions, avoid making unnecessarily strong solutions and rinse and dry the hands after exposure. The longer the solution, or any residue of it, remains in contact with the skin the more chance of irritation developing.

**Question:** What exactly is eczema and what are the vitamin additions and deficiencies connected with this condition?

**Answer:** Eczema is defined as a disease of the skin characterized by inflammation, itching and the formation of scales. It is not chronic and can be treated rather quickly. A diet deficient in needed fatty acids can produce eczema. Conversely, people with small amounts of essential fatty acids in their blood have been prone to the disorder. Treatment required to clear up eczema would be the addition of vegetable oils to the regular diet. Soy bean oil in particular is good. In regard to children, eczemas appearing soon after birth are caused by mothers avoiding fats during pregnancy, being unaware of their own need for linoleic acid, which has been shown to help prevent or cure eczemas resulting from a lack of any one of the several B vitamins. This is probably because this fatty acid stimulates the growth of intestinal bacteria which can produce these vitamins. Particularly a lack of B vitamins—PABA (Para-amino benzoic acid) and B6 results in eczema appearing first in the scalp and the eyebrows, in the nose, behind the ears and around the genitalia. Too much of one B vitamin can also cause havoc. Often the B complex tablets are heavily into one particular B supplement, deficient in others such as pantothenic acid. It has been shown that people taking a large amount of B-complex tablets daily had only increased their need for what was lacking—pantothenic acid, vitamin B6, PABA and/or biotin a lack of any one of which could cause eczema.

**Question:** Please give me some background into the skin disease known as psoriasis.

**Answer:** Psoriasis is the chronic skin disease characterized by scaly, reddish patches on the skin. It is a disorder for which a cause is not readily known. It is the positive suggestion that psoriasis is a disease involving incorrect use of fatty foods by the body. Although recommendations for treatment consist largely of salves, ointments and compresses, psoriasis is a disease involving chiefly incorrect diet. Hence it should be easily preventable and perhaps easily cured by proper diet.

What are these elements of diet? First, the fat soluble vitamins —that is, the vitamins which exist and are soluble in fats and oils, rather than those soluble in water. The fat soluble vitamins are vitamins A, D, E, K and those mysterious substances we are just now investigating which some researchers call vitamin F—the essential unsaturated fatty acids. Also, certain of the B vitamins are necessary in the diet if the body is going to use fatty substances properly. Pyridoxine and nositol, are necessary in the digestive tract if we are going to digest and use properly the unsaturated fatty acids. Chronic means lasting a long time or recurring. Occasionally, the disease will pop up in people who are taking the proper amount of vitamins and adhering to the rules of fine nutrition. That is why its exact origins can prove a puzzlement to physicians. But the diet approach is still the best thing we have and psoriasis sufferers would be wise to try soybean lecithin along with vitamins A and D and the following B vitamins: thiamin, pyridoxine, ribloflavin and pantothenic acid. The kind of fat you bring into your system is most important. Of course, there are plenty of inexpensive fats around to eat. But it is not the quantity, but the quality that is of major concern. Fats occur naturally in many foods of animal and vegetable origin. Seeds are our chief source in the vegetable kingdom—grains, nuts, sunflower seeds, etc. Butter, milk, eggs and fat meats are sources in food of animal origin. From our vegetable fats our refining processes have removed much that is of value nutritionally—especially lecithin and the B vitamins that go along with nature. White flour lacks these valuable substances. Also corn oil, peanut oil and so forth are hydrogenated these days. This is a chemical process destroying the unsaturated fatty acids most essential for good health. Shortenings used for frying and baking are hydrogenated as is margarine and commercial peanut butter. The recommendation is to eat little "fatty food" of any kind. Those you do eat should be all natural fats—eggs, salad oils, sunflower seed, avocados, raw nuts. Eat your meats, poultry and fish broiled or roasted, without gravy. Eat plenty of fruits and vegetables, and avoid desserts which, with their heavy sugar and white flour, rob you of the B vitamins. If one is to combat psoriasis, synthetic fats must be eliminated.

**Question:** How does an ordinary pimple develop on a person's face?

**Answer:** The lack of vitamin A causes cells in the lower layer of the skin to die and slough off. They plug the oil sacs and pores, thus preventing oil from reaching the surface; the skin becomes dry and rough and sometimes the entire body itches. The pores plugged with dead cells cause the skin to have the appearance of "goose pimples" although they are unaffected by temperature changes. Pores enlarged by an accumulation of dead cells and oil are spoken of as whiteheads or blackheads. If these cells become infected, pimples may very well result. The skin is likewise susceptible to such infections as impetigo and boils. These abnormalities can usually be corrected by increased amounts of vitamin A, provided the diet is adequate in other respects.

Many people involved in doing office work, usually under

fluorescent lights and naturally with the continuous use of their eyes, together with the glare and reflection from white paper, have a greater need for vitamin A which is involved in successful day and night vision. Also A is sensitive to light and eyestrain and this simultaneously allows abnormalities to occur in the tissues spoken of as mucous membranes. During a vitamin A deficiency the cells of the mucous membranes grow more rapidly than usual but quickly die. These cells are crowded forward by other rapidly growing cells which likewise die until there accumulates a cheesy-like surface of layer upon layer of packed, dead enzymes, their surface is no longer washed and their self-protective mechanisms are gone. Heat, moisture and a replenished food supply combine to set up conditions for bacterial growth: bacteria themselves are ever present. Infections—pimples—are usually the result.

**Question:** A black friend recently suffered the disappearance of natural color, in patches and blotches on his face. I've been told this skin condition is called "vitiligo" and would like to know more about its causes and treatment.

**Answer:** Vitiligo is a painless skin disease which is character-ized by the disappearance of natural color, or pigment, from patches on the skin. Even the fairest skins have some color, and when it goes, these patches of absolute white are very definitely visible and can be most embarrassing. In a darker skin the prob-lem is emphasized. An absence of free hydrochloric acid in the stomach has been known to cause vitiligo asserting the important part that diet plays in curing this condition. Also hormonal imbalance can cause the disease. Contributory factors are wounds, infection, pressure points and light rays. In some cases the addition of the B vitamin PABA has cured vitiligo through injections as well as tablets as the vitamin alone taken orally does not remain in the bloodstream for a sufficient length of time to act effectively. In most instances the dietary deficiencies must be fully corrected, hormonal inbalances righted and local infections cleared up before a single vitamin can be expected to have any effect. The B complex as it appears in brewer's yeast, desiccated liver, wheat germ and the organ meats, would seem essential in preventing the occurrence of vitiligo.

**Question:** Exactly what brings on itching of the rectum?

**Answer:** Itching of the rectum—technical name, pruritus ani—is a very likely location for contact dermatitis. Not only are the sources of contact more numerous than one would imagine (soap, clothing, toilet tissue, enema nozzles, suppositories, orally administered antibiotics which have passed through the digestive system and laxatives) but the area is moist and covered, so that germs and fungi have an excellent breeding ground. The foods we eat which pass out of the body undigested, in fecal matter, might also cause a reaction with the tender skin of the rectum. This is especially true of such hot foods as mustard, horseradish and pepper. Moisture is constantly present in the rectal area due to a system of sweat glands which are part of the sexual glandular system. These glands are highly responsive to emotion or sexual tension, so that an emotional or sexual state can cause perspiration which can lead to itching. Few people can resist scratching and this added irritation only causes a worsening of the condition. Effective treatment of this condition is based on these general principles: keep the area clean by careful removal of all fecal matter, but do not use soap or toilet tissue, for both of these should be avoided. The use of clear tap water is best. Then dry with cotton or a soft, clean cloth. Do not scratch through clothing, as harmful dyes are readily introduced in this way. White underclothes should be worn to lessen the possibility. The area should be kept as dry as possible and no ointments or greasy salves should be used.

**Question:** Can you give me a brief summary—a catchall of rules to follow to maintain healthy and beautiful skin?

**Answer:** Your skin is an eliminative organ and when it is unable to function properly, poisons are retained in the system and this leads to an impure bloodstream and general ill health. Restore healthy skin functioning with wholesome natural foods and sound natural hygienic care as discussed in preceding questions and answers regarding skin condition and care. Stay away from artificial and concentrated sweets and starches. Exercises also do much to rebuild the functioning of the skin. The hot baths are of great help, while a good friction rubdown with a brisk brush or a turkish towel brings a glowing feeling of warmth to the skin and promotes more normal functioning.

## BIBLIOGRAPHY

Bronson, Barnard Sawyer, *Nutrition and Food Chemistry*, J. Wiley & Sons, Inc.

Clark, Linda, *Secrets of Health and Beauty*, Pyramid Books.

Cummings, Richard Osborn, *The American and His Food*, University of Chicago Press.

Davis, Adelle, *Let's Eat Right to Keep Fit*, Signet Books.

Davis, Adelle, *Vitality Through Planned Nutrition*, Macmillan Co.

Flatto, Edwin, *The Restoration of Health—Nature's Way*, Pyramid Books.

# THE KIDNEYS

**Question:** What is the function of the kidneys and are they a large part of the relationship between the heart and blood vessels?

**Answer:** The kidneys are part of a special unit, with the heart and blood vessels, that together controls circulation and affects the health of the entire body. While the heart acts as the pump that maintains the circulation and the arteries provide the channels through which the blood circulates, the kidneys are the organs that filter the toxic wastes from the blood. Another important function of the kidneys is to control the fluid content of the body. About two thirds of the human body is composed of fluids. The cells contain fluids and live in a fluid medium. The blood, also, is largely composed of fluids. Fluid is taken into the system with our food and drink, and has to be eliminated when it is not able to be used by the body. Some of it is expelled through the lungs in the form of vapor when we exhale. We excrete some through our sweat glands, but the greatest portion is usually eliminated through the kidneys. The kidneys have an elaborate filter system composed of miles and miles of hair-sized filtering tubules. In one day many quarts of fluid pass through these filters, but the greatest amount is reabsorbed by the tubules and only about one to two quarts are actually eliminated through the kidneys. When the kidneys become damaged, they are unable to filter out the wastes from the blood and the intricate mechanism that controls the fluid content of the body is unable to function efficiently. This upsets the equilibrium in the body and places an increased burden on the heart and the blood vessels. How important the function of the kidneys is to the maintenance of health can be seen from the fact that approxi- mately 20 percent of all the blood pumped by the heart is carried to the kidneys. When the heart is damaged, the kidneys fail to re- ceive an adequate supply of blood and this in turn impairs the intricate filtering mechanism and upsets the fluid balance. As a result, fluids begin to accumulate in the system, appearing first in the area of poorest circulation, the feet and legs, and then, as the disease progresses, in the abdomen and chest. The retention of this fluid places an added load on an already overworked heart and may ultimately progress to the point where the patient virtually drowns in his own fluids. It should be apparent that the kidneys are so very closely related to the heart and blood vessels, the damage to one organ will adversely affect the function of the others.

**Question:** What exactly is meant by the condition of kidney stones and is it still prevalent in the United States today?

**Answer:** A century ago, kidney stones were an important cause of illness especially among young people. Today kidney stones are far less prevalent in this country and the emphasis as well has shifted from youth to age. Today, kidney stones seem to be a disorder of older people who are lacking in the essentials of good nutrition. No one knows exactly how or why the stones are formed, but it is generally agreed that diet plays a part. One possible cause of stones could be related to a high content of oxalic acid in the diet, as the stones appear to be formed chiefly of calcium oxalate. Foods such as spinach, chocolate and cocoa contain lots of oxalic acid which also causes the body to lose calcium. Also, vitamin deficiencies contribute to the formation of stones. The effect of vitamin A on the cells lining various passages in the body such as the urinary passage is well known and an adequate amount of the vitamin must be ingested in order to keep the urinary mucous membrane in good condition. Urinary stone occurs frequently following ulcer therapy and the dietary restrictions involved. Also, it is contended that the lack of vitamin C directly affects the urinary tract, wherein the mucus lining scales off and forms the nucleus of the stones. Cloudy urine containing phosphates (which constitute some kinds of kidney stones) and pieces of sloughed off mucus from the walls of the urinary canal went hand-in-hand with vitamin C deficiency. Giving large doses of vitamin C could clear the urine within a matter of hours. There is a hypothesis that contends that stone is a deficiency disease, with vitamin starvation acting primarily on the lining of the kidneys and through it on the colloidal mechanism of the urine; once the mechanism is deranged, stone formation must follow as a direct result of the laws of physical chemistry. This is an interesting statement, obviously with a basis rooted in fact, but as we said earlier, no one knows exactly how or why the stones are formed.

# THE LIVER

**Question:** What of the liver and its supposedly many functions in the body?

**Answer:** The liver is considered the jack of all trades in our body, serving many functions. And a vigorous, normally performing liver is one of the best protections against disease.

The liver is one of our most essential organs. It plays a vital role in the digestion and assimilation of food, as well as in the elimination and/or detoxification or neutralization of the toxins of the body. Some of the functions of the liver illustrate the role it plays in the maintenance of our health and well-being. It manufactures the bile essential for the digestion of fats. When the liver is unable to secrete enough bile the fats are not completely digested, and this can lead to many serious ailments. Fats not fully digested tend to deposit a film of fat on other foods, and they too become more difficult to digest. This explains in part why it is recommended that no butter be used with potatoes or bread and why it is advisable that in cooking the use of fat be greatly restricted or even completely eliminated. The bile also prevents putrefaction in the colon and by accelerating peristaltic action helps to regulate bowel functioning. Another function of the liver is to modify the digested protein foods and prepare them for assimilation by the cells and the tissues of the body. The liver also completes the break-up of the starches and sugars, and stores the final product, in the form of glycogen, for future use, releasing it only when the body requires it for fuel and energy. When the body is deficient in sugar, the liver (under certain conditions) can convert protein and fat into sugar. The liver also acts as a vast reservoir for vitamins, minerals, and enzymes, and even manufactures some of them when the needs of the body are great. It converts the carotene of carrots and other yellow vegetables into vitamin A and stores many of the other vitamins and minerals for use when needed. Finally, one of the most essential tasks of the liver is to neutralize and render harmless the many irritating substances and toxins that accumulate in the body as a result of the metabolic processes, or are taken into the system with our food and drink or in the form of chemicals and drugs.

**Question:** Since a complete breakdown of the liver would mean death in less than two hours, what is the best way of keeping this organ healthy?

**Answer:** Nutrition is just about the very best protection of the liver. The implication is this: if liver disease is present, only nutritional therapy is effective; if one would avoid liver trouble, be sure to maintain good nutrition. A solid supply of B vitamins must be present, plus plenty of vitamin C and other vitamins and proteins, and one should avail oneself of organ meats for possible vitamin factors not yet defined. Equally important is the avoidance of those items which might rob the system of the B vitamins already there. Both smoking and alcohol are known to do this. And smoking is especially destructive of vitamin C. In the case of the liver, lack of vitamin C apparently causes the same condition that this deficiency causes in other parts of the body. The intercellular material begins to dissolve and collapse. Giving vitamin C immediately causes the liver to begin to reconstruct these cells once again. If you are getting plenty of vitamin C there is far less chance that you are going to develop hardening of the arteries with all its accompanying effects on the heart and the blood vessels. And there is far less chance that whatever fat you eat is going to collect in the liver to do perhaps deadly damage there. Choline, part of the B vitamin group, is very important for liver health. Choline prevents livers from becoming "fatty" so it is spoken of as a "lipotropic" substances, that is, something which is attracted to fats and hence is useful in helping the body manage them properly. Regarding proteins, a diet containing ample complete protein is essential for liver health. Most foods (except white sugar) contain some protein. But you need complete protein—that is, protein in which all of the essential amino acids or forms of protein are present in the right proportions. Foods of animal origin provide this almost exclusively. It is difficult to arrange a good high protein intake on a vegetarian diet. It is impossible on a diet in which there are refined carbohydrates. You need 60-70 grams of complete protein a day. And if you want to keep the liver healthy avoid synthetic vitamins. They're dangerous, especially as you may get overdoses of some which will throw the level of others out of balance. Get your vitamins from natural food sources, like brewer's yeast, desiccated liver, fish liver oils and rose hips.

**Question:** What is the disease known as cirrhosis of the liver?

**Answer:** Cirrhosis of the liver is a major cause of death in the United States. And although exactly what causes the disease is still unknown, about one-fourth of the deaths from cirrhosis of the liver are reported to be associated with alcoholism. Certainly the disease, in general, is related to alcohol intake.

First, let's look at what happens physically when cirrhosis sets in. The liver becomes hardened and infiltrated with scar tissue. The damaged parts of the liver, at first, become greatly enlarged, but later begin to shrivel up and waste away. At this stage, the liver is usually very hard and small, sometimes as small as half its natural size. When the liver is enlarged, this condition is known as hypertrophic cirrhosis, while when the liver shrivels up and wastes away, it is known as atrophic cirrhosis.

The relation of alcoholism to liver disease is an obvious one. The alcoholic subsists mostly on carbohydrate, for alcoholic beverages are pure carbohydrate. Furthermore, the appetite has been so perverted by alcohol that the alcoholic sometimes goes for long periods of time with no food at all. Then, too, for the body to handle the pure carbohydrate of alcohol, B vitamins must be provided, for they are an essential part of the metabolism of carbohydrates. They are practically nonexistent in the alcoholic's diet, so they are stolen from his body—nerves, muscles, brain tissue and digestive tract. Another good reason for liver trouble dogging the steps of the alcholic. Several of the B vitamins are of the utmost importance to the health of the liver—especially choline and inositol, two B vitamins most concerned in the handling of fat by the body. We know also that harm to the liver comes from eating too much of the wrong food. Cirrhosis of the liver is a widespread disease in parts of the world where there is little animal protein in the diet; that is, the people eat largely carbohydrate diets. And it does not seem to matter how fine a source of carbohydrate they may have or how natural all the foods are. If the animal protein is lacking, cirrhosis of the liver is most likely to occur. So many people seem to try to get along on little or no protein—that is, eggs, meat, poultry or fish. Here, particularly in the United States, where there is plenty of animal protein available, cirrhosis of the liver has now climbed to tenth place among diseases that kill. Look at the people about you who have a cup of coffee for breakfast, a sticky bun and a cup of coffee for lunch and perhaps only a couple of grams of protein for dinner. According to the official recommendation, children should have from 40 to 100 grams of protein every day. Adults should have from 60 to 70 grams. There are certain poisons in our environment that are peculiarly damaging to the liver. Anesthetics are one. Several of the antibiotics are known to be poisonous to the liver when they are taken by mouth and injected at the same time. Other poisons considered destructive to the liver are: chloroform, bromide, arsenic and antimony, cinchophen, picric acid, poisonous mushrooms, and carbon tetrachloride. It seems impossible, with our present knowledge, that anyone would be exposed to these poisons to such an extent to harm the liver. But do we know how much harm may be done to the liver by small doses of these over a long period of time? Arsenic, for instance, is widely used in insecticides of which a residue is bound to stay on the fruit. How much must accumulate in the body before damage is done to the liver? We are not certain. Bromides are used in sleeping pills and sedatives. The number of such medications taken in our country every year is almost astronomical. What relationship does it have with the rising incidence of cirrhosis of the liver? Other diseases may contribute to liver trouble. Impaired digestion, such as ulcerative colitis which brings about such a deficiency in many valuable food factors that the liver cannot continue to function properly. A lack of appetite can bring about the same condition. An overactive thyroid may burn up the abnormal amount of food and thus deprive the liver of badly needed elements. Disorders of other glands may have the same effect. We have talked about cirrhosis of the liver at length because this is the most serious liver disease one can have, the one most likely to be fatal, the one most likely to lead to cancer, the one that indicates the most serious disruption of orderly body processes. In general, however, what we say about preventing cirrhosis of the liver applies to other liver disorders as well. If you keep your liver healthy you are not going to take to your bed with any of the diseases mentioned. And it is surprising how much agreement there is among authorities as to the best safeguard for the liver. Medical opinion is practically unanimous. What you eat and do not eat and what poisons you are exposed to—these are the important factors in liver health.

**Question:** What of hepatitis, which suddenly seems to be a common disease in the neighborhood. My son who is a college student tells me there are people in his class coming down with hepatitis. I was not aware that it was all that common and even infectious. Can you tell me more about it?

**Answer:** Hepatitis is one of those cyclical diseases which are on the rise for a few years, then subside for a while, only to flare up again. However, even in its wildest rampages, hepatitis never made such a showing as the current one. We know that hepatitis is caused by a virus which has yet to be isolated, and therefore scientists can only guess at how the virus is transmitted, how long it will stay, what damage it will do and if the disease will recur. There are two types of hepatitis: infectious and serum. Infectious hepatitis is thought to come to the victim through food, water, bodily contact, etc. The serum hepatitis virus is conveyed by way of transfusions and injections given directly into the bloodstream. When hepatitis does occur, the virus can remain in the blood system for as long as 5 years before making itself known by its classic symptoms. When it does take hold, hepatitis is first characterized by a gradually increasing weakness and dizziness which appears to many to be the first stages of grippe or a bad cold. Soon utter and complete fatigue occurs along with nausea, pains in the stomach, tenderness in the liver area and an unconquerable loss of appetite. The urine is noticeably darker in color, the virus acts to destroy the tissue of the liver, and interferes with the liver's ability to process waste materials of the body. The skin and the whites of the eyes take on a yellowish tinge due to the escape of bile pigments into the blood and tissues. The seriousness of this attack on the liver can be gauged by the fact that this organ is responsible for the manufacture of important blood components and the storage and processing of certain vitamins. It must eliminate poisons which come into the body through polluted air, insecticides and pesticides, sprayed on foods, chemicals in processed foods and drugs. If it is not functioning, all of these elements pile up in the body and can poison the entire system. Fortunately the liver is able to restore itself, if given the proper nourishment. The trouble is that hepatitis victims are always short on appetite, and find it difficult, if not impossible, to eat the food they need so that the liver has something to work with in its repair operations. Injections of B vitamins are sometimes given to aid in nourishing the liver. No definite treatment for hepatitis seems to have been devised. For many years it was believed that prolonged bedrest was essential. Current thinking has the patient up and about as soon after the initial attack as he feels able, as comparison has shown that neither course has any effect on the length of the illness. Diet-wise, the victim should use natural fats and avoid hydrogenated fats and fried foods. Eggs, for example, while high in cholesterol, are rich in lecithin which helps to use the cholesterol properly. They are also rich in the B vitamins which are essential to the liver's good health. Food supplements are recommended as one should always be aware that with sufficient nutrition the liver would have never been susceptible to such a violent attack in the first place.

Hepatitis virus of the infectious type is largely propagated by unsanitary conditions. It can be spread through polluted water systems and through contaminated foods. The virus is known to survive sewage, and flies can carry and spread the virus. The more sensational type of hepatitis, serum, has really made the headlines in recent years. A visit to a doctor or dentist for treatment of an illness, or for some preventive measure might result in infection with an even worse illness, hepatitis. Hepatitis is easily transmitted in injections, even if platinum needles are used and flamed after each injection. The only way to eliminate the risk of inducing hepatitis by inoculation is to use a newly sterilized needle and syringe for each injection. Disposable needles are one answer, but complete sterilization of all the implements the doctor uses, especially those which puncture the skin, should be the rule. The most effective defense against the spreading of hepatitis is extreme care in sanitation. Particularly since the possibility of the disease spreading within families is great. More than one case per house is not uncommon. Keeping things clean, concentration on vitamin-rich foods and avoidance of any others which might induce a weakness in the liver. This warning especially applies to liquor. Be sure of your water source. Bottled spring water is best. Aside from these, effective precautions against hepatitis are scarce. Gamma globulin injections can be given to those who think they have been exposed, but there is no such thing as a hepatitis vaccine. The gamma globulin is a serum rich in antibodies which is believed to help the body fight infectious viruses when they attack. Unfortunately any protection that might come with this serum is temporary. Also, one who is injected with this preventive measure should be certain that all precautions against serum hepatitis have been taken, lest one be injected with the disease rather than the preventive.

**Question:** I have recently heard of a condition known as "biliousness" in reference to the liver. Is this a disease and does it have anything to do with food intake and digestion?

**Answer:** Consider "biliousness" a disorder which at one time was regarded as a disorder of the liver, but is now thought of as an outgrowth of constipation. It shows up when there is an increase in the secretion and a backing up of bile. Constipation, loss of appetite, coated tongue, bad taste in the mouth, headache, dizziness, nausea and occasionally, extreme pain in the pit of the stomach, with vomiting and fever, usually accompany it. Treatment requires that all food be stopped. And when nausea or vomiting is present, even water should be withheld. If necessary, an effort to induce vomiting artificially is often helpful to cleanse the system. Two tablespoons of ordinary table salt dissolved in a glass of lukewarm water, followed by two glasses of plain cold water, should be swallowed quickly, immediately after the salt solution has been taken. This solution sometimes washes down the irritating material and provides relief in that way, but in the majority of cases it will cause an emptying of the stomach by vomiting. After the acute symptoms have subsided small quantities of easily digestible bland foods may be introduced. Raw or stewed fruits for breakfast, and small meals composed of grated raw and plain steamed vegetables for the noon and evening meals. Fat foods, spices, stimulants of every kind and processed and refined foods must be strictly excluded.

## BIBLIOGRAPHY

Abrahamson and Pezet, *Body, Mind and Sugar*, Holt, Rinehart, Winston.

Bourne, Geoffrey, *Biochemistry and Physiology of Nutrition*, Academic Press.

Bragg, Paul, *Toxicless Diet Body Purification and Healing System*, Health Service Co.

Fraser Harris, P., *The Man Who Discovered the Circulation of Blood,* Popular Science Monthly Pub.

Nuzum, Franklin Richards, *The Span of Life As Influenced By the Heart, the Kidneys and the Blood Vessels.*

Warmbrand, Max, *The Encyclopedia of Natural Health*, Groton Press.

Weston, Drake, *Guidebook for Alcoholics: How to Succeed Without Drinking*, New York Exposition Press.

Williams, John Roger, *Alcoholism: The Nutritional Approach,* University of Texas Press.

# THE GALLBLADDER

**Question:** I know that the function of the gallbladder is to store the bile, which is secreted by the liver. But what happens if the gallbladder becomes diseased? How is the bile thus treated?

**Answer:** Not only does the gallbladder, which is a pear-shaped organ attached to the undersurface of the liver, store the bile, but it also empties it into the small intestine whenever it is needed. Unlike the liver, in which a great deal of inflammation and deterioration can often exist for long periods of time without any apparent discomfort, an inflammation of the gallbladder is usually accompanied by a great deal of pain and suffering. In a diseased gallbladder, many destructive changes can take place. An inflamed gallbladder usually becomes distended and swollen, and tiny hemorrhages and ulcers often develop. As the inflammation continues, the walls of the gallbladder become thickened and filled with scar tissue, and its power to contract and empty the bile diminishes and ultimately may be completely lost. An inflammation of the gallbladder may occur as an outcome of disturbances in the gallbladder proper, or may develop as a result of disturbances in the bile duct or in any other organ close to the gallbladder or the duct and can cause interference in the drainage of the bile. when the bile becomes stagnant in the gallbladder, it gradually begins to change. The solid elements begin to crystallize and gravel and stones begin to form. The liquid portion, too, undergoes disintegration, changing to substances that vary from a bile-stained loose fluid to thick pus. Many factors lead to an obstruction in the bile duct. The duct may become obstructed when long-standing irritation causes its tissues to harden, destroying its ability to stretch and relax. It also becomes obstructed when, following a previous inflammation, scars or adhesions have formed. Particles of mucus that get into the bile duct as well as pressure from adjacent organs that have become inflamed or enlarged also cause pressure on the duct and interfere with the outflow of bile. Stones in the gallbladder may also obstruct the duct and cause an interference with bile drainage. In a case of this kind, however, the

50

presence of a previous inflammation that has given rise to the formation of stones may be assumed. Long-standing irritation of the gallbladder by toxins carried to it by the bloodstream is another factor that plays a part in the onset of inflammation of the gallbladder and/or bile duct, and leads to the formation of stones. These toxins are present in the bloodstream either because the liver has been unable to destroy them or render them harmless, or because the kidneys or other eliminative organs have not been able to expel them. A frequent cause of gallbladder inflammation is a derangement in the chemical makeup of the bile or a high concentration of cholesterol. These chemical disturbances are usually the outgrowth of faulty nutrition and incorrect living habits and are often brought on by an impairment in the metabolism of the body. A high concentration of cholesterol in the gallbladder often goes hand in hand with a high cholesterol content in the blood.

**Question:** What exactly are gallstones and what is the cause of them?

**Answer:** A gallstone by definition is a small, solid mass sometimes formed in the gallbladder or bile duct, and it can obstruct the flow of bile, causing a painful diseased condition. Since the chemical imbalance in the bile is not always the same, the stones that develop in each case are not always of the same type. Some stones may be formed only of a concentration of cholesterol, others only of calcium or of some of the other solids, while others may be a composition of the different solids of which the bile is composed. This is the reason why stones do not always show up equally well on the X-ray plate, and why soft stones made up primarily of cholesterol often do not show up at all, when fully formed. The size of the stones also varies considerably. Some may be very small, even of the pinpoint variety, while others may be very large. In some cases, the gallbladder may contain a great many stones of various sizes.

Cholelithiasis is the medical name for gallstones, and many possible causes for them have been mentioned down through the years. There seems to be no doubt that the formation, for one, of gallstones is intimately related to diet. Those who have trouble with their gallbladders are usually overweight. This means, of course, that they overeat. Or that they eat more than they should of certain foods. Usually, too, they are over 40, although recently more and more cases of gallbladder trouble are occurring in younger people. The flow of bile may be obstructed in cases of overweight people and pregnant women, where the actual weight of the fleshy tissue stops off the flow of bile in the little ducts. This causes it to back up into the gallbladder, and trouble ensues. Then, too, it seems that gallstones may be caused by what is called "disturbed metabolism" of cholesterol. Cholesterol is a fatty substance that exists in fatty foods of animal origin. Most gallstones contain cholesterol and it seems obvious that the stones would not have been formed in the first place had not something gone wrong with the way the body is supposed to use cholesterol. Apparently the amount of cholesterol in the diet has little to do with the formation of stones. Yet the favorite diet given to gallbladder patients for relieving gallstones is a cholesterol-free one. It is known that the materials that go to produce gallstones are made when your body burns fat. The way your body burns fat depends on your glands. The amount of fat it has to burn depends on your diet. The vitamins in a diet are of the utmost importance to the way the body uses fat. Both choline and inositol B vitamins are involved with the ability to transport and digest fats and cholesterol to the various fat deposits in the body. And biotin, another B vitamin, is directly involved in the assimilation of fat by the body. It must be present in the intestine in ample quantity or fat cannot be digested. Also, the fat soluble vitamins (A, D, E and K) must be considered when you are planning a diet to prevent gallbladder trouble. They are present in fatty foods, and if you should decide to go on a low-fat diet to prevent gallbladder trouble, you are likely to run into serious difficulty because you will simply not get enough of the fat soluble vitamins. And vitamin K is directly affected by anything that goes wrong with the gallbladder. Bile must be present in the intestine or vitamin K cannot be absorbed by the body. Vitamin K is responsible for the proper coagulation of the blood. Could a lack of vitamin K caused by gallbladder disorder be partly responsible for today's tragic incidence of cerebral hemorrhages or "strokes?" There seems to be evidence that this is indeed true. And we are told that a lack of vitamin A can affect the lining of the gallbladder.

We have now begun to hear about vitamin C and its connection to gallstones. Vitamin C is absolutely necessary for the health of tissues. It must be present to form the cement that holds cells together. When there is not enough of it, cell material flakes off and forms a kind of garbage which has no place to go. In the genitourinary tract these provide the nucleus for kidney stones which bring a certain amount of infection and begin to collect layers of other material around them. This vitamin C theory is just that in regard to gallstones, but since vitamin C is just about the most important single item in everybody's diet, regardless of health, why not give the theory a try? There is nothing to prevent you, and you could become healthier from it.

**Question:** Can you tell me of the care prescribed during an acute gallbladder attack? And is it true that gallstones can dissolve or disintegrate, thus preventing surgery?

**Answer:** This question would best be answered in two parts. First, one can take a look at gallbladder attack which may be brought on when a stone itself gets into the duct and interferes with the free flow of the bile. In these cases measures must be employed to relax the duct in order to give the stone a chance to pass through. Medically, opiates are used for this purpose, but they often have a disturbing and harmful effect upon the body. It is recommended to use simple, natural methods which, when properly applied, accomplish the same ends, but leave no bad after-effects. As soon as an acute attack sets in, it is imperative that all food be discontinued and that only hot water be taken, plain or flavored with a few drops of lemon or lime juice. This will help to flush the system. Also the use of frequent enemas to clean out the bowels and hot baths to induce relaxation are most effective. Hot, moist compresses applied over the gallbladder regions are often of great help. These measures must be continued until the acute attack has been completely subdued. It is true that opiates usually provide relief more rapidly, but since they leave the body considerably weakened and subject to recurrent attacks, we prefer to rely upon this simple natural approach. In addition, the measures suggested help to lay the foundation for improved health. After the attack has subsided, the abdomen may continue to be sore and sensitive, but this will diminish with each passing day and will usually disappear within a week. This type of care has been instrumental in saving thousands of gallbladder sufferers from needless surgery. However, to attain lasting results it is imperative that this program be carried out with the aid of a physician and most consistently in accordance with the particular needs of the case.

Regarding gallstones and dissolution or disintegration, it is believed that if the above program is applied consistently and the body's metabolic functions are gradually restored to normal that stones often dissolve and disintegrate. Those formed of the softer substances, such as cholesterol, usually disappear more rapidly, but even those formed by the harder substances will often break down, although much more time may be required before results are attained.

## BIBLIOGRAPHY

Albanese, Anthony August, *Protein and Amino Acid Nutrition,* Academic Press.

Bacharach, Alfred Louis, *Science and Nutrition,* Watts and Co. (England).

Duncan, Garfield G., *Diseases of Metabolism,* W. B. Saunders Co.

Fredericks, Carlton and Goodman, Herman, *Low Blood Sugar and You,* Constellation-International Pub.

MacLeod, Florence, *Fat-Soluble Vitamins and Calcium in Nutrition,* Columbia University Thesis.

Rodale, J. I. and Staff, *The Encyclopedia of Common Diseases.* Rodale Books, Inc.

Wattles, Wallace D., *Health Through New Thought and Fasting,* Health Research Pub.

Warmbrand, Max, *The Encyclopedia of Natural Health,* Groton Press.

# COLDS

**Question:** I have a large family—six children—and find that a cold is a common occurrence in my household. What is it exactly that causes a cold to develop?

**Answer:** A cold happens when the mucus membrane of the nasal passages and/or the other organs of the respiratory system have become inflamed and irritated by toxic waste products that have accumulated in the system, and must be eliminated. A healthy body must always discard its toxic waste products. When the body does become overworked or exhausted or when it becomes overloaded with too many of these toxic by-products, the organs of elimination—-the nose, the kidneys, lungs, skin and intestines—are unable to cope with all the work. Result: an excess accumulates in the system.

**Question:** My husband and I recently moved up north to be with our children and grandchildren. All our lives we had lived in Florida and had been proud of the fact that our children and ourselves rarely came down with a common cold. Now in the new environment we find that our children, grandchildren—even ourselves, are coming down with all sorts of cold infections. Is the change in climate a major factor?

**Answer:** In this case the obvious is very true. Cold weather is an important aspect in the cause of colds. Many doctors in keeping records of children in various climates have correlated the number of cold infections with the daily temperature. Extreme cold brings a "potent stress factor" which lowers the body's resistance and brings about a cold within 9 to 12 days. As person after person in the community gets the cold, they establish immunity and by the time the winter weather is over, the epidemic is over. You should realize that this cold weather explanation is not an end in itself. Certainly people come down with summer colds and there are cold germs bothering individuals in warm climates. But it is

55

likely that the chilling northern weather is always accounting for the susceptibility to cold infection.

**Question:** Is vitamin C really effective in protecting against common cold germs? It seems everywhere you go, all you hear about is vitamin C and the common cold.

**Answer:** Look at this example to begin with—"In a cold climate for man to survive, the lower the temperature, the more vitamin C is required." This relationship of vitamin C to cold weather is only the beginning. Yes, vitamin C is an excellent preventive of colds. Perhaps many of us suffer from frequent colds for two reasons: first, we are not careful enough to choose foods that initially contain vitamin C and second, we may not know how to preserve the vitamin C in foods until the time we eat them. Vitamin C is the most perishable vitamin there is. It is lost when foods are stored or cooked. It seeps away into the water when foods are soaked. Get all the vitamin C you can. It can't possibly harm you. Fresh fruits and vegetables all year round would supply you with that needed vitamin. Remember that vitamin C is necessary in the fight against any infection, including cold infections. At the sign of a sniffle, you should begin to take massive doses of natural vitamin C. Colds are shortened and made much less serious and troublesome if you take natural vitamin C preparations from the start, straight through the course of the cold. Any excess which your body does not need will be excreted harmlessly. Being that vitamin C is important to your health, you should make every effort to prevent colds, rather than trying to cure them, by supplying enough of this vitamin to your system at all times.

**Question:** A neighbor recently told me that feeding a large amount of wheat cereal to my family could possibly stimulate colds. Is there any truth to this?

**Answer:** Cereal contains a high amount of carbohydrates. A high intake of carbohydrates disposes one to upper respiratory problems, such as colds. Carbohydrates tend toward water retention in the body and persons with stuffed noses are, of course, described as having an excess of water in the body. Controlled studies of pupils of a girls' boarding school who were fed a quantity of foods with lots of sugar—including cereals—were compared with children whose diets had a minimum of sugar. It was found that the group with the lowest rate of sugar consumption had less amount of colds, percentage-wise.* Inflammation of mucus membranes of the body was markedly higher with a diet consistently rich in carbohydrates.

**Question:** I recently went to a family physician with the complaint that one cold followed another this past winter and this was happening in spite of a healthy diet full of necessary vitamins. He diagnosed a lack of calcium and prescribed accordingly. What exactly is the correlation between calcium deficiency and the common cold? I never really understood the connection.

**Answer:** This to the average public is not common knowledge, but the correlation between calcium and cold prevention can be answered rather scientifically. In the nose, there are little, almost microscopic hair-like things called cilia, which cover the mucous membrane and which move forward and backward like a field of wheat in the wind. They are as close together as the hair on a rug. They move the secretions of the nose into proper channels. They are easily affected and then either function poorly or not at all. The cilia need calcium for "backbone" to stand up to their job, and since a terrific percentage of the public is calcium deficient, you can see how the lack of calcium in one's system can court realistic trouble as far as colds are concerned.

**Question:** Could you tell me just how important vitamin A is in preventing cold infection? Also, what foods are prime sources of this vitamin?

**Answer:** Vitamin A does not directly kill germs, but it does preserve the normal physiological functions and structure of the mucous membranes. It also aids in the regeneration and restoration of these membranes in the event they become injured or destroyed. To understand the actions of vitamin A in cold prevention, we once again turn to discussion of the cilia. Cilia, located on the surface of the normal mouth, bronchial membrane and the

*British Medical Journal quoted in *Encyclopedia of Common Diseases* by J. I. Rodale and Staff.

nose, sweep foreign matter, including germs, toward the pharynx where it can be spit up or swallowed. In an individual who is not getting or absorbing enough vitamin A, a change takes place in the mucous membrane. The cells with cilia gradually disappear and are replaced by scaly, hard cells, which do not have cilia. The substances secreted by the membranes are cut off and the dryness increased. Thus, when the germ comes along, there is no defense against it. Although the action by this vitamin against colds is an indirect one, it is a major one. The preservation of the strength and health of the cells of the mucous membrane, and also the rejuvenation and replenishment of these cells when they have been destroyed or injured by attacks of germs, are believed to be vitamin A's function regarding cold prevention.

You ask about foods, and the following all contain large amounts of vitamin A: fresh calf and beef liver, carrots, dandelion greens, whole eggs, endive, lettuce, parsley, turnip greens, water cress, spinach, green peppers, sweet potatoes, tomato juice and of course, fish liver oils, the latter containing many times more vitamin A than any other food.

**Question:** I tend to salt all the food I serve, three meals a day. Recently, I had a bad cold and I was advised by friends to stay away from salt. Why is this so?

**Answer:** It is very possible the use of a salt-free diet would minimize the occurrence of common colds. The chemical content of table salt is sodium and chloride. The chloride serves no purpose in our bodies except that it may go to form hydrochloric acid in the stomach, a certain amount of which is necessary for digestion of proteins. An excess of salt in the diet can result in too much hydrochloric acid in the stomach, which will surely produce stomach ulcers. It is the sodium part that pertains most specifically to colds. To a certain extent, sodium cancels out the necessary functions of calcium. Sodium chloride tends to liberate calcium. Impairment of the calcium function will only lead up to possible inflammatory effects.

**Question:** I read somewhere that garlic is a remedy for the common cold. That it is better than aspirin which I've been told can destroy vitamin C in the body. Why garlic? Is there any truth to this or is it an old wives' tale?

**Answer:** Why not give a natural remedy like garlic a chance. Yes, there is truth to its effectiveness. Down through the ages of man, particularly in European societies, garlic has been talked of as being suitable as a remedy for many types of infectious diseases, including clogged and running nose, cough and sore throat. The oil of garlic is composed in part of sulphides and disulphides. These unite with virus matter in such a way that the virus organisms are inactivated so their harmful effects cease. All of this is done without any danger to the healthful organisms in the body. Therefore if you do enjoy the taste of garlic, there should be no reason why you would not seek to make use of this healthy bulb in your diet. It definitely does inactivate harmful viruses!

**Question:** I have heard people talk of the psychological aspects of colds; that a person's feeling under the weather because of mental strain can make him more susceptible to cold germs. Is it true that nervousness and tension can cause colds?

**Answer:** It is known that any state of stress or anxiety is known to cause shallowness of breathing, which to many ways of thinking is the most frequent cause of nasal congestion. Excitement and tenseness make correct breathing difficult. But it is because of that breathing difficulty that one must learn to relax the body's tenseness. Consciously deep breathing relieves lots of anxiety. And just remember that it is almost impossible to breathe deeply and "Be nervous" provided that your nose is not too badly blocked.

**Question:** Please in the shortest, most concise definition tell me what influenza is, and what the average person can do, at home, to cure this disease in the quickest way possible.

**Answer:** Influenza is a simple disease that usually responds easily to proper care. Call influenza, "an acute, infectious fever affecting the mucous membranes of the body," for this is what it is. Now know that there are rules to follow if one is to prevent the disease from turning into a more serious, highly complicated disorder.

You should plan on a complete rest in bed and, of course, the elimination of all foods except diluted fruit juices or hot water flavored with lemon juice. The intake of important vitamins is, of course, essential. Now additional treatment, not often known to the average person, should be incorporated. You should use warm water cleansing enemas for the first few days. Then these enemas can be eliminated as normal bowel action is restored and the acute condition is brought under control. Also the use of hot epsom salt baths, once or twice a day, with the patient returning to bed immediately after the hot bath. Not to be overlooked as well is the application of cold compresses, (not ice) to the forehead to keep the head cool, and a hot water bottle or heating pad to the feet to keep them warm. All this should be administered in a room that is well ventilated. And you should be aware that quiet and lack of excitment are also prime ingredients in getting rid of influenza.

**Question:** In combating a cold, I have heard that it is wise to eliminate as much solid food as possible from my diet, in order to recover rapidly. Is this true?

**Answer:** This is very true, indeed. In fact, if you are after the most effective care for colds, you should start by eliminating *all* solid food. This is done to cut down the work of the digestive organs and to provide them with a resting period. This also lessens the burden of work for the eliminative organs, and gives them a chance to catch up with their work. Orange juice, grapefruit juice, grape juice, apple juice, hot lemonade sweetened with honey, or hot vegetable broth is permitted. Yes, by all means avoid solid food.

**Question:** What about the use of "a shot of penicillin" to get rid of a bothersome cold?

**Answer:** We have come upon a great deal of information on harmful reactions to penicillin among hospital personnel who are not taking the antibiotic themselves, but have been so exposed to it while they were giving it to patients that they are now extremely sensitive to it. Of course, the rest of us do not come in contact with the antibiotics every day. But what proof do we have that a dose of penicillin from time to time—for a cold, for a cut finger or for almost anything else—may not in time make us sensitive, too?

Attention has been called to the fact that the severity of reactions to penicillin, currently being administered as a last-minute cure-all in the treatment of even non-infectious complaints, is greatly increasing. Whereas previous sensitizations produced by the drug had resulted principally in skin eruptions, such as itching, nettle rash and hives, the list of newly observed post-injection effects now includes prostration, symptoms of arthritis, shock, chills, and fever. All require protracted periods of readjustment for recovery, which may be marked by still further irritations. Resistant strains of disease organisms are appearing that have acquired immunity to the antibiotic drugs, such as penicillin and aureomycin. Continued misuse of the drugs will increase the number of resistant strains. All these drugs do is to halt the growth of germs which the body's natural defense mechanisms then destroy. The usefulness of the drugs depends therefore on the condition of the patient, his state of nutrition and his general stamina. If the natural defense is at a low stage, the antibiotics are not apt to help much. Also, it is believed that antibiotics in powder or ointment form are probably of little benefit, and the combined use of several antibiotics together appears to be of little value.

**Question:** I've heard that people who smoke a great deal have a definite susceptibility to colds. Is that true?

**Answer:** It is known that smoking is harmful. Smoking cigarettes exposes your lung and throat tissues to tobacco tar containing benzopyrene. And the ugly, greasy tar that is left in the ashtray, on your fingers or in the filter of your cigarette holder is not nicotine. It is the "soot" that is left from the incomplete combustion of the tobacco—just as dangerous as the soot from your chimney. Also, the way you smoke has something to do with how much injury you may encounter. The way you puff your cigarette, how long you hold the smoke when you inhale, how far down the butt you smoke your cigarette, all these have some bearing on how much irritation you are subjecting your throat tissues to. Rapid smoking, for instance, causes more irritation, because the smoke enters the mouth at a higher temperature. There is a definite disease known to medical science as "smoker's asthma," a condition with cold symptoms brought on by smoking. "Smoker's asthma" is a chronic inflammation of the Adam's apple area of the throat: wheezing, shortness of breath, a tendency to respiratory infections, constriction of the chest above the heart and prolonged coughing in the morning, sometimes requiring several hours to clear the throat of mucus. Physicians should always make allowance for the possibility of "smoker's asthma" when they are diagnosing ailments. Smoking uses up vitamins that protect us against colds and other disorders—especially vitamin C and vitamin B. So, we can see here, that the smoker, aside from irritating his nose and throat membranes, at the same time deprives them of food elements that might help to protect against these poisons. Considering the fact that his respiratory membranes are pretty constantly in a state of irritation, is it any wonder that, when the cold bugs attack, they find good pickings in these depleted, sick membranes? The weapons that might defeat them have already been used up and the smoker becomes easy prey for the sniffles, the tears, the fevers, the chills, the coughs, the hoarseness and, perhaps, finally, pneumonia.

**Question:** I understand that shallowness of breathing is a most frequent cause of nasal congestion. I am often plagued by this congestion and wonder if you have any suggestions on how to clear up this condition.

**Answer:** First, examine whether or not you are the type of person who walks around tense a good deal of the day. If so, this might be the reason for the difficulty in breathing correctly. It would be wise to learn to breathe correctly. This will work in a kind of little circle as correct breathing will relax the body's tenseness. You will find that it is almost impossible to breathe deeply and be on edge, provided that your nose is not too badly blocked. Consciously deep breathing also relieves anxiety. We can offer a little breakdown here of good breathing exercises. a) Breathing must be as deep as possible without undue strain. b) Breathing must be through the nose only, unless the nose is so completely blocked as to preclude the passage of air. In this event, inhale through the mouth and exhale through the nose, until the nose is clear enough to permit inhaling through it. c) Breathing must be at a pace slow enough to avoid tiring. d) Breathing for the purpose of opening each side of the nose must be persevered in until it is completely open. e) Head posturing (that is, placing the head, during the breathing exercises, in positions that will favor the drainage of the sinuses under the force of gravity—usually reclining) should be resorted to from the start. Perseverance is important to success in these exercises. Every hour, each side of the nose must be checked to make sure that it remains open. If either side has become blocked, the exercises must be resumed and continued until the nose is completely opened again, no matter how long it takes.

**Question:** My neighbor is constantly overdressing her children. Even in rather mild weather they are in sweaters and coats. Is there an automatic cold connected with overdressing?

**Answer:** Overdressing seems to be a problem imposed on civilized man by the conventions of a society whose purpose it is to sell, sell and more sell. Overdressing, of course, can produce a cold in your system. A body thus prohibited from ridding itself of excess heat, and even adding extra warmth, is leaving itself wide open to colds and sickness. Too many people suffer the discomfort of clothing that is impractical, because society may dictate that the particular item should be worn. Today, in our country, because of the psychological demands placed on dressing, we can see truth in the visualization of the sweltering male who, in winter, is bundled up in tweeds in a house kept warm enough for women's low cut dresses and chiffons, and in summer must wear jackets and ties in public, when the weather clearly dictates the loosest and lightest of minimal attire.

**Question:** Once my cold seems to be over, is there any special vitamin pill, taken in strong dosages and continuously, that would prevent another cold from coming on?

**Answer:** The dosage of certain vitamins, as has been previously discussed, will help cure common colds, but it should be remembered that it is even more important to be aware of the prevention of colds as your main goal. And this must be done through maintaining a healthy, balanced metabolism through good day-to-day, healthy living. After your cold has been conquered, the adoption of a well-regulated diet, composed of wholesome natural goods, along with adherence to sound health-building measures, will be sure to strengthen your body and establish an optimum state of health. Talking about just one vitamin in excessive dosage is talking about "pill magic," and that is something best saved for the storybooks.

BIBLIOGRAPHY

Alsakar, M.D., Rasmus, *Conquering Colds and Sinus Infections,* Groton.

Bottemly, H. W., *Allergy: Its Treatment and Cure,* Funk and Wagnalls.

Clark, Linda, *Get Well Naturally,* Arc Books, Inc.

Davis, Adelle, *Let's Get Well,* Harcourt, Brace and World.

Hessler, Robert, *Colds and Cold,* Indiana Academy of Science Press.

Rucker, William Colby, *Common Colds,* Government Printing Office, Washington, D.C.

Shelton, Herbert M., *Health for the Millions,* Health Research Pub.

Townsend, James Gayley, *A Review of the Literature on Influenza and the Common Cold,* Government Printing Office, Washington, D.C.

Williams, Richard G., *Health Culture for Busy Men,* Cassel and Co. (England).

# PNEUMONIA

**Question:** When one contracts pneumonia, what stages does the inflamed lung or lungs go through?

**Answer:** Before entering into a discussion of pneumonia, it should be explained at the very beginning that the many misconceptions about the disease in the lay public's mind have to do with the success of modern-day treatment. By this we mean that people have come to believe that pneumonia can be overcome with modern antibiotics in therapy that takes a matter of a few days. However, this is not really true. No real case of pneumonia is completely overcome unless the massive inflammation that exists in this disease is completely eliminated. The antibiotics often suppress fever and the other symptoms of this disease, but this does not necessarily mean that the disease has really been overcome. In pneumonia, what happens specifically is that there is an extensive, massive inflammation of the lung with a severe degree of toxemia or poisoning, and fever. At the onset of the disease the affected part or parts of the lung become inflamed and congested and start pouring out a thick sticky substance that fills up the soft spongelike air spaces in the lung. This sticky substance causes the affected part or parts of the lung to solidify and take on the appearance of a solid organ like the liver. However, because the solidified parts of the lung are engorged with blood, the color at first is red. In about four or five days, the red color changes to gray. By this time, the solidified substance that filled up the air spaces has become even harder, and the lung is heavier than ever.

**Question:** Are there different types of pneumonia and, if so, what are the symptoms indicating the particular affliction?

**Answer:** This disease usually has been classified into various types, but there are really only two major forms: bronchopneumonia and lobar pneumonia. Bronchopneumonia develops gradually, and usually shows up as a complication of influenza, bronchitis, measles, whooping cough, or even the common cold. In this type, only patches or spots of the affected lung are involved. Lobar pneumonia usually develops suddenly. Lobar pneumonia's onset is marked by chills, fever, coughing, chest pains, and shortness of breath. Nausea, vomiting, diarrhea, and headaches also often accompany Lobar pneumonia. This type of pneumonia differs from bronchopneumonia in that the inflammation will involve a whole section or sections at once, rather than just spots. Recovery varies with the case. In some cases, health returns by a gradual clearing up of the symptoms. In Lobar pneumonia, however, the change is often sudden and dramatic. The patient may seem to be in grave peril and yet within a few hours may have passed the critical stage and be on the road to recovery. Various complications increase the dangers in pneumonia. In some cases, resolution of the solidified mass may be incomplete; in others, the lung tissue may break down; while in some, purulent matter or considerable pus may form. The latter is the condition known as empyema. Pericarditis, an inflammation and thickening of the covering of the heart, and otitis media, an inflammation of the middle ear, are some of the other serious complications that may develop in relation to pneumonia. And pleurisy is known to be present in almost all cases of pneumonia and will tend to intensify the patient's suffering.

**Question:** Can you tell me about treatments administered originally to sufferers of pneumonia? Are these treatments still in prominent use?

**Answer:** To determine the type of treatment that is best it is imperative that we investigate the results that were obtained with the different forms of treatment that have been used in the last fifty years, and compare them with the results that can be obtained when measures are employed that aim at promoting detoxification, the rebuilding of bodily resistance through proper nutrition, and the restoration of the body to its normal state. The treatment of pneumonia has gone through a transformation. At the turn of the century, treatment in pneumonia was directed primarily to the control of symptoms. This was known as supportive treatment. Aside from the use of oxygen, which is a great need in some cases, the remedies then prescribed included narcotics to induce sleep and make the patient comfortable, and medicines to reduce fever, relieve pain, ease the cough, and support the heart. Using narcotics and other suppressive drugs, in the old days, may have made the patient more comfortable and/or masked the other symptoms of the disease, but actually suppressed the defensive mechanism of the body. This deprives the patient of his only weapon to overcome pneumonia. This explains why so many of these cases developed serious complications, and why the mortality in those early years was so high.

Then, the introduction of serum therapy eliminated the use of many of the suppressive drugs and brought about a reduction in mortality. The sulfa drugs followed, but they caused many toxic side effects, and were ultimately replaced by the antibiotics. Today, pneumonia is treated primarily with antibiotics, although some doctors use the sulfa drugs as well as antibiotics. There is no question that the replacement of mass medication by the antibiotics brought about a considerable reduction in mortality. It is well to stress at this point that antibiotics have no curative effect. They inhibit bacterial action and thereby check some of the symptoms of the disease, but the congestion still exists and the disease is not overcome until the material that has filled in to the air spaces and has become solidified is finally resolved and absorbed. It is important that we realize that although antibiotic therapy is an improvement over previous treatments, it also acts as a suppressant and thereby interferes with the defense mechanism of the body, and this is undoubtedly the reason why the mortality, although materially reduced, is still frightening. Doctors are becoming increasingly aware that antibiotics interfere with the defense mechanism of the body. Controlled experiments have demonstrated that patients with pneumonia who are given a chance to develop their own natural immunities are much more comfortable during their illness, do not develop as many complications, and usually recover much more rapidly. Those cases, on the other hand, in which antibiotics have been used from the very beginning of the disease are usually subject to relapses, often develop serious complications, and usually take much longer to get well. The hazards of antibiotic therapy have been recognized for a long time, and proof of these dangers has been mounting at a rapid rate. Rushing in with the antibiotics or any other antibacterial drugs often complicates the situation, since these remedies inhibit or destroy the favorable micro-organisms and, undoubtedly, other living entities necessary to the maintenance of life and health, such as the enzymes, and possibly even our own cell structures. It has been known for some time that the antibiotics, by inhibiting or destroying the favorable intestinal bacteria, lay the foundation for a great many serious intestinal disorders. The fact that they interfere with the body's efforts to cope with the disease by building up its own natural immunity is but another of their many evil effects, and only increases the danger in these cases. When the sulfa drugs are used in addition to the antibiotics, the risks are only multiplied. No wonder this type of therapy in pneumonia, although less life-destroying than the previous treatments with mass medication, still produces a frightening mortality.

**Question:** If suppressive drugs and serum therapies are not the answer in treatment of pneumonia, what today is to be recommended for recovery?

**Answer:** We've seen already that drugs were most destructive because they interfered with the defensive mechanisms of the body. We therefore must look towards methods of treatment which will not interfere with the body's defense mechanism, and will provide successful results. At the onset it is important to realize that good nursing is essential in the treatment of this disease. The patient must be kept quiet and relaxed, both physically and mentally, must be kept warm and comfortable, and must be protected against overexertion. The sickroom must be well ventilated and must be kept clean and quiet. The patient should be supplied freely with fluids. Hot or cold water whenever desired, plain or flavored with lemon juice, and diluted fruit juices are soothing. No solid food should be allowed during the acute phase of this disease. Constipation must be controlled. Daily enemas are a great help for this very purpose. Where the patient is not too weak, hot baths twice a day, for a few minutes at a time, are of great help. Following the baths, the patients should be wrapped in cool wet packs. These packs improve circulation, promote elimination through the skin, and make the patient more comfortable. The packs are left on for one to one and a half hours. The patient is then sponged off with tepid or cool water and made comfortable. Where the patient is too weak for the full baths, hot mustard baths may be used, and the moist packs should then be applied. Cool spongings also help to make the patient more comfortable. For greater comfort, the patient may be propped up in bed; his position should be changed frequently. In severe cases, oxygen may be necessary, and is often of great help. This program, adjusted to the individual case, is carried on until the congestion has been resolved and the patient is out of danger. Patients with some influenzal or borderline types of pneumonia may recover within a very few days. A massive type of lobar pneumonia, however, has to run its full course of consolidation, hepatization, and resolution, before it is completely overcome. In some cases of bronchopneumonia only small patches of spots may be involved, and cases of influenza or acute bronchitis may sometimes be mistakenly diagnosed as pneumonia. While these cases may respond quickly, they do not represent the pattern that is to be expected in the more massive types of pneumonia.

**Question:** What about the general diet and nutrition rules to follow while coming out of a pneumonia condition and immediately following recovery?

**Answer:** As we've mentioned, when being treated for pneumonia the patient should be supplied freely with the proper fluids. Hot or cold water whenever desired, plain or flavored with lemon juice, and diluted fruit juices, are soothing. No solid food should be allowed during the acute phase of the disease. Then, immediately following recovery, a bland diet composed of the wholesome natural foods should be gradually introduced to rebuild the patient's health and vitality. It should also be noted that recent studies of certain pneumonia cases, resulting in death, have found evidence of serious vitamin A deficiency and the case histories of the patients involved revealed either of two things: they had not obtained enough vitamin A in their diets or because of some digestive disorder, such as liver trouble or diarrhea, they had not assimilated whatever vitamin A they obtained. The evidence regarding vitamin A and just how it prevents infection has been of a conflicting nature in relation to pneumonia.

# BRONCHITIS

**Question:** Is bronchitis simply a disorder which manifests itself as a cough?

**Answer:** When the inflammatory condition of an acute cold or acute sinus condition extends into the bronchial tubes, we have what is known as acute bronchitis. In this condition, there are severe and sudden attacks of coughing as well as high fever, due to the inflammation and swelling of the trachea and bronchial tubes. Large quantities of sticky, stringy, mucus are usually expelled. There are cases, however, where the cough is dry and little or no mucus is brought up. In these cases, the sudden attacks are usually more severe and more debilitating. It is well to stress at this point that a cough is an effort on the part of the tissues to loosen up and expel irritating material, and that as such it must be regarded as part of the defensive mechanism of the body. It should not be suppressed. To overcome the irritating and annoying cough the toxic or irritating substances must be eliminated, and the inflammation must be overcome. This can be accomplished most effectively when measures are employed that improve the circulation and increase the functions of the other organs of elimination, such as the kidneys, skin, and intestines. The program outlined for the acute cold, or sinusitis, is therefore also applicable in acute bronchitis. It is well to point out though that an acute bronchial disorder may take somewhat longer to overcome than the simpler respiratory acute ailment and that, therefore, more patience and perseverance may be required.

**Question:** What makes for the condition of chronic bronchitis and why does it continue to persist?

**Answer:** Sufferers from chronic bronchitis usually have histories of frequently recurring colds, acute bronchial attacks or other acute respiratory diseases. Chronic bronchitis is rather common among individuals past fifty or sixty years of age. It is common for people with rheumatic and kidney diseases, heart disease,

70

obesity and other chronic ills. Excessive intake of alcohol and the use of tobacco are other causes. Sometimes the affliction is due to irritating substances inhaled with the air supply, such as irritating gases and excessive amounts of dust. The word "chronic" means lasting a long time and this is the important definition to keep in mind in effecting treatment. When a program of diet and physical care is initiated to rid the sufferer of chronic bronchitis, the measures taken, in some cases, may lead to the onset of one or even several colds. This is not an indication that the patient is getting worse, but that the acute condition that has been suppressed is now reawakening and that the toxins and irritants that have accumulated in the tissues and caused the existing damage are breaking up and being eliminated. These reactions are merely nature's effort to convert the chronic ailment into an acute state, and should therefore be welcomed, since this is the way the body usually overcomes its chronic ailments.

**Question:** What is the best treatment for a chronic bronchitis condition?

**Answer:** The treatment for chronic bronchitis involves essentially the same procedure as any other chronic catarrhal (inflammation of a mucous membrane) condition. The circulation must be improved, the elimination of toxins must be promoted, and the general health of the body must be rebuilt. This requires a bland non-irritating alkaline diet composed primarily of raw and steamed vegetables, raw and stewed fruit, plus moderate amounts of proteins, and the use of easily digestible vegetable carbohydrates such as the root vegetables and/or baked or boiled potatoes. Fat foods, refined and processed flour and sugar products, refined cereals, coffee, tea, spices and condiments must be eliminated. These foods cause an acid residue that is highly irritating and provide little or none of the needed protective elements. Dairy products too are inadvisable in these cases and should be avoided or greatly restricted. Whenever possible, complete abstinence from food, or at least from solid food, for a limited period of time is highly advisable. An abundance of rest and sleep, hot epsom salt baths, and deep breathing, as well as other moderate physical exercises are of great help in these cases. When a program of this kind is initiated, improvement usually begins at once. The discharge of mucus may first increase, but before long is greatly reduced; and ultimately dries up completely. The sudden attacks of coughing gradually diminish in severity and, in time, are completely overcome.

Many people ask about change of climate in curing the condition of chronic bronchitis. While this move may do some good, the disease is really caused chiefly by autointoxication, which is mostly based on wrongs of digestion and elimination. That's why proper diet as stressed above is the key to clearing up the entire condition.

## BIBLIOGRAPHY

Baker, Henry Brook, *The Causation of Pneumonia*, Michigan Health Board Reprint.

Bottemly, H. W., *Allergy: Its Treatment and Cure*, Funk and Wagnalls.

Clark, Linda, *Get Well Naturally*, Arc Books, Inc.

Copper, Lenna Francis, *Nutrition in Health and Disease*, Lippincott.

Glynn, Ernest Edward, *Bacteriological and Clinical Observations on Pneumonia and Empyemata*, Oxford University Press (England).

Rodale, J. I. and Staff, *The Encyclopedia of Common Diseases*, Rodale Books, Inc.

Young, Matthew, *The Influence of Weather Conditions on the Mortality from Bronchitis and Pneumonia*, Journal of Hygiene (England).

Wattles, Wallace D., *Health Through New Thought and Fasting*, Health Research Pub.

Warmbrand, Max, *The Encyclopedia of Natural Health*, Groton Press.

# THE SINUSES

**Question:** Whenever I hear the word sinus, I think of my nose. But could you tell me the exact relationship between the two in physiological terms?

**Answer:** The sinus can most easily be defined as a hole in the head, except that we actually have many holes and therefore we speak of sinuses—not a sinus. The sinuses are the hollow spaces or cavities in the bones of the head, surrounding the base of the nose. They help to lighten the bony structure which would otherwise be quite a burden to carry around. In addition, they act as sound boxes for the voice. The vocal cords might be compared to the strings of a violin. The sinuses, then, are like the spaces enclosed in the violin proper in which the sounds reverberate. The sinuses are arranged in the head in a particular order. The sphenoid sinuses are a pair of sinuses high up and toward the back of the nasal passages. The openings from these sinuses point almost directly forward. In front of them and slightly below are the posterior ethnoid sinuses which drain inwardly toward the nasal septum, the partition which separates one nasal passage from the other. There may be a half dozen or more of these posterior ethnoid sinuses. In front of them lie the anterior ethnoid sinuses which drain mostly in an outward and downward direction. Both anterior and posterior ethnoid sinuses lie in the ethnoid bone about the middle turbinate (another bone). Near the anterior ethnoid openings are the openings of the frontal sinuses and antra. The frontal sinuses lie in the forehead above and between the eyebrows and their openings point downward, while the antra lie in the face under the eyes and drain upward into the nasal passages. In all, we find an average of fifteen or twenty nasal sinuses in the normal head. Some open outward, some up and some down. What all the names and locations boil down to is that all these various holes are grouped about your nose, and drain, one way or the other, into your nasal passages.

**Question:** What happens to the sinuses in the condition known as sinusitis?

**Answer:** The openings from most of the sinuses into the nasal passages are no bigger than the thickness of the lead in a pencil. The secretions that accumulate when one has a cold are thick and gummy. They can't get through. We were meant to clear the sinuses of mucus by blowing our noses. Air can be blown forcibly through the nasal passage, and it is blown over the fifteen or twenty individual sinus openings, if the nasal passage is normal. The passage of air creates suction which draws the liquid up so that it can be expelled by the air. So in the normal nose it is easy to empty all of the sinuses simply by the nose. Hence many people never have any trouble at all with their sinuses and don't know what it means to suffer the excruciating pain of sinusitis. The sinusitis sufferer is a victim of obstructed nasal passages for one reason or another and so fluid secretions collect in his head. The pressure of the fluid is what makes the pain. Someone whose nasal passages are narrow may be able to keep them well drained most of the time. But when a cold comes along and the mucous membrane inside his nasal passages swells, fluid may accumulate and sinusitis may develop. If you have a well-formed and healthy nose, you probably won't have sinus trouble. If you were born with nasal passages that are too narrow to perform their function, or if you have suffered from a blow on the nose, chances are that you have or may develop sinusitis. Normally blowing one's nose clears all secretions from the sinuses, for, as the air passes over the sinus openings, the suction created draws the fluid out into the nose. However, if the passages of the nose are too small to accommodate the air, or if some injury to the nose has closed up those passages, the mechanism will not work and secretions begin to accumulate in the sinuses. Then, too, when you get a cold the potentials of severe sinusitis starting are more prevalent as the mucous membrane of the nose swells and may shut off the nasal passages altogether. This is known as chronic sinusitis and it often gives rise to polyps forming and a great deal of scar tissue developing. A constant postnasal drip is a symptom in these cases.

The nasal membrane is extremely sensitive to all kinds of

influences which could relate to the development of sinusitis. A little loss of sleep, cold or wet feet or a draft at the neck may be all that is necessary to cause the membrane to swell and become congested. Many people even have some nasal congestion after a heavy meal. In head colds, the inflammation spreads along the mucous membrane so it causes more mucus, which produces pressure inside the sinus. The accumulated fluid becomes coagulated, thick and gummy. When there is enough of this fluid to overflow, it is forced out into the nasal passage, but the sinus is by no means drained. If the nasal passages are too narrow, or swollen with congestion from the cold, the rest of the mucilaginous matter remains in the sinus and causes more and more irritation.

**Question:** What prevention methods or treatments besides operations can relieve sinus conditions.

**Answer:** I'm glad you said "besides operations" because it is known that operations for sinus conditions are not notably successful. When surgeons make new openings into the sinus cavities, the bones and cartilage tend to grow back together, so the project fails and the sinus fills up with fluid once more.

It is well to keep in mind how important diet is in the formation and maintenance of well-formed mouth and nasal passages. Prospective mothers can assure their children of good bone formation by eating diets in which refined foods are reduced to a minimum and vitamins A and D are plentifully supplied, as well as calcium and the other important minerals. Too much white flour and white sugar in the American diet from childhood on has been known to change the bone structure within one generation. Teeth become crowded, the dental arch is small and narrow and noses take on a narrow pinched look. The one symptom that seems to be present in all patients with colds and sinus infections is acidosis, meaning the patients have not been getting enough of the alkaline-forming foods in their diets. And one of the early symptoms of vitamin A deficiency is lowered resistance to colds. Vitamin A is necessary to maintain the tissues in the skin of the body and the linings of body openings, such as the throat and nose. The mucous membrane in these linings is known to dry up considerably during the early stages of a cold. Protein from the animal foods—meat, fish and poultry, are of course, important to a good diet. But it is well to remember that these foods are acid-forming in the body and must be balanced with foods that have an alkaline reaction. These are, in general, the fruits and vegetables. Also, sufferers from colds and sinusitis should keep to rye bread, graham bread and pumpernickel whenever possible. All of the cereals used should be unrefined. Sugar is another evil which should be omitted entirely from the diet to avoid colds and sinusitis. Not eating salt, or doing so at a minimum, from the point of view of sinus trouble is explained by its relation to calcium in body metabolism. If large amounts of sodium chloride are taken, a good deal of it will be stored in the skin, mucous membrane and other tissues, and calcium will be liberated. Therefore, each sodium molecule retained in the tissues will diminish the calcium effect. And this is important in preventing colds and other inflammations of the nasal passages. To prevent colds and sinus trouble, the diet should be "salt-poor"—not more than 5 grams of salt per day.

For immediate local relief of pain, the application of heat to the back of the head and cold moist compresses (not ice) over the forehead is recommended. In some cases the use of hot, moist compresses over the forehead has a more soothing effect, and is therefore to be recommended in preference to the cold compresses. After the acute stage is overcome, the carefully regulated nutritional program we mentioned above, and adherence to a sound program of living, will rebuild the vitality of the patient and protect against recurrences.

BIBLIOGRAPHY

Alsaker, M.D., Rasmus, *Conquering Colds and Sinus Infections,* Groton Press.

Bourne, Geoffrey, *Biochemistry and Physiology of Nutrition,* Academic Press.

Carrington, Hereward, *Vitality, Fasting and Nutrition,* Rebman and Co.

Davis, Adelle, *Let's Eat Right to Keep Fit,* Signet Books.

Shepard, John Frederick, *The Circulation and Sleep,* Macmillan Co.

Sweetzer, Rodney, *A Look at the Condition of the Sinuses,* Lippincott.

Ullman, Egon U., *Diet in Sinus Infections and Colds,* Macmillan Co.

————, *The Secret of Sinusitis and Headaches,* Liveright.

# THE PROSTATE GLAND

**Question:** I think most people are confused as to what the prostate gland really is. I know I think of it as being closely related to the male sex organ, but I am not certain. What exactly is the prostate gland and how can one tell that there is trouble brewing in that area?

**Answer:** Before even looking at the symptoms, as you suggest, we should give a brief education regarding location and function of the prostate gland. The prostate gland is located near the mouth of the male bladder. The gland itself functions as an auxiliary sex gland. It manufactures the liquid which acts as a vehicle for the sperm cells of the male. Without the important fluid there is no way of transferring the sperm into the female vagina for the purpose of fertilizing the female egg, and hence no way of carrying out the normal process of reproduction. Without the prostate gland to manufacture this essential fluid the male becomes sterile. When the prostate becomes swollen or enlarged it invades the area occupied by the urethra. This is the tube through which the urine is expelled from the bladder, and the swollen prostate gland pressing upon the urethra interferes with the normal flow. The complications which result can be frightening and most painful. In the early stages, the symptoms of enlarged prostate are rather vague: a feeling of congestion and discomfort in the pubic area. There follows a constant feeling of fullness in the bladder, with frequent, urgent trips to the bathroom. Once there, there is often difficulty in starting a stream, and sometimes no urination at all. The recurring need to void during the night is also common. Eventually, a residue of urine that has not been expelled is collected in the bladder and dribbling occurs. This is the unconscious release of urine, in small amounts, forced out by a full bladder. When the urethra is interfered with to the extent that very little or no urine can escape from the bladder, the serious problem of possible uremic poisoning arises. This can occur when such large amounts of fluid accumulate that the bladder can hold no more. With the normal

78

avenue of release through the urethra shut off, the urine floods back into the kidneys, presenting a grave danger of poison to the system.

**Question:** Are there particular treatments now in use that deal with prostate problems?

**Answer:** There are several courses of treatment. Perhaps with the condition of an enlarged prostate, attention must be paid to the immediate relief of a full bladder. For this a catheter is employed. Usually it consists simply of a sterile rubber tube which is inserted into the urethra and gently pushed along its length to the mouth of the bladder. The bladder empties through the tube quickly and with ease. This method is excellent for emergency treatment, but not for constant repetition. For one, it is extremely painful, and the chance for infection as well as damage to delicate tissues is very real. For another, the bladder fills quickly, and catheterization would have to be maintained almost daily if relief were to be consistent. Finally, this is no more of a solution to the cause of the problem than to give a man standing over hot coals injections of morphine to kill the pain instead of making him get off the coals.

Another means of relieving the symptoms of swollen prostate is to massage the gland. This can be accomplished by a physician and is often effective in reducing the swelling. But the treatment must be repeated about once a week. So-called sitz baths in which one soaks only the lower portion of the trunk have a soothing effect and often reduce the swelling, but are obviously inconvenient. The average doctor's final opinion on what to do about prostate trouble is to have it removed. The operation has come to be reasonably safe and relief is sure. Of course, sterility is an inescapable aftermath of the operation, though this does not mean that there is any lessening in the patient's desire for sexual activity. The person who has had his prostate gland removed is perfectly normal in this respect, but for the fact that he can't father a child. It is understandable, however, that men are anxious to find some other way to solve the prostate problem.

**Question:** Are there particular nutritional approaches in recent years that have been employed to relieve enlarged prostate?

**Answer:** If the prostate swelling is simply a benign condition of enlargement, then the non-surgical treatment using a nutritional approach is most realistic. Recently, an amino acid compound with a mixture of three amino acids (kinds of protein)—glycine, alanine and glutamic acid—had resulted in a patient's urinary symptoms disappearing and enlarged prostate returning to normal. However, the patient remained free of the symptoms while taking the compound, but soon after discontinuing the medication, the symptoms returned.

Other nutritional elements employed include the use of vitamin F, or the unsaturated fatty acids. Treatment with the unsaturated fatty acids resulted in a more complete emptying of the bladder, with an increase in sex urge and a lessening of fatigue and leg pains. Though there are no formal experiments on record, there are two vitamins which should have a beneficial effect in the prevention and treatment of prostatic disorders—vitamin A and vitamin E. It is known that a deficiency of vitamin A shows up first in a sloughing off of the cells which line the digestive, respiratory and reproductive tracts. This indicates a weakness of the cells which make up the structure of these important organs, and serves as a warning that nutrition to these parts is lacking. Weakness such as this serves as an excellent breeding ground for trouble. Your vitamin A supply should be carefully maintained. Aside from its demonstrated effectiveness in treating heart conditions and other illnesses, vitamin E is generally accepted as an effective agent in maintaining the health of the reproductive tract. Wheat germ oil, high in vitamin E, is considered to be effective in preventing reproductive disorders. Scientists hazard the guess that natural hormones which occur in wheat germ oil are partly responsible for its good effect. These elements should be in one's diet at all times. For a man faced with the danger of prostate trouble to chance being short of vitamins A, E, and F (unsaturated fatty acids) and the amino acids found in protein foods, would really be tempting fate. Foods high in these 3 amino acids—alanine, glutamic acid and glycine—are those foods which are richest in protein. Soybeans and peanuts are extremely valuable sources. You should make it a practice to eat more of these foods.

**Question:** What is the new theory on treating prostate gland disorders which has to do with using pumpkin seeds in the diet?

**Answer:** Dr. W. Devrient of Berlin is a German doctor who recently announced a new theory concerning pumpkin seeds in regard to prostate gland troubles. Dr. Devrient believes that the seeds contain materials which are the building stones for the male hormones. Thus they are actually supplying the body indirectly with the means of carrying on the work of the male hormones. In certain countries where pumpkin seeds are eaten in great quantity throughout life, there is almost no incidence of enlarged prostate or other prostate disorders. Quoting Dr. Devrient: "Only the plain people knew the open secret of pumpkin seeds; they all knew that pumpkin seeds preserve the prostate gland and thereby, male potency. In these countries (Hungary, Bulgaria, Ukraine) people eat pumpkin seeds the way they eat sunflower seeds in Russia: as an inexhaustible souce of vigor offered by Nature. My assertion of the androgen-hormonal (the male hormone) influence of pumpkin seeds is based on the positive judgment of old-time doctors, but also no less on my own personal observations throughout the years. This plant has scientifically determined effects of intermediary metabolism and urination, but these latter are of secondary importance in relation to its regenerative, invigorative and vitalizing influences. There is involved herein a native plant hormone which affects our own hormone production in part by substitution, in part by direct proliferation."* A number of different substances have been found to be contained in pumpkin seeds, but no one has ventured a guess as to which it may be that brings about the good results on the sex organs. We do know that they are extremely high in phosphorus and low in calcium (as are most seeds). Their iron content appears to be higher than that of any other seed. The B vitamins are plentiful, as they are in other seeds, and there is a small vitamin A content. They contain about 30 percent protein and about 40 percent fat. The fat, of course, is rich in unsaturated fatty acids, as are most vegetable fats. Perhaps these are the responsible agents in pumpkin seeds. And what of the protein content? It seems quite possible that the protein content of pumpkin seeds, along with the unsaturated fatty acid

*Encyclopedia of Common Diseases* by J. I. Rodale and Staff.

content, may be responsible for the seed's reputation as a regulator of sex organs. Perhaps the best recommendation of all for the pumpkin seeds may at the same time be the explanation for the lack of prostate disorders in parts of the world where the seed is widely eaten. Pumpkin seeds are a completely natural food. Their fat and proteins are unchanged and untampered with. They provide in good measure all the rich nutriment that the plant needs to germinate and to grow.

**Question.** What of special zinc deficiency and the enlarged prostate gland?

**Answer:** The normal prostate gland contains more zinc than any other organ in the body. Sperm cells, processed by the prostate gland, contain more zinc than any other part of the gland. These facts were turned up rather recently and several researchers have been doing further study on them. What do they mean from the point of view of the health of the prostate gland? Is it possible that a deficiency in zinc in the diet might be at least partly responsible for trouble with the prostate gland? Zinc is a trace mineral—that is, a mineral which exists in very small amounts that can just barely be "traced." It has been found to be an important part of a body enzyme, "carbonic anhydrase." This enzyme takes an essential part in conveying carbon dioxide in the blood and is also concerned in some way with the body's acid-alkaline balance. All of these mechanisms would be considerably hindered if the body lacked zinc. In laboratory experiments, it has been found that a diet lacking in zinc causes some of these changes in animals: decrease in growth, hair that does not grow properly, spots around the mouth like those of patients suffering from vitamin B deficiency, changes in the eyes caused by vitamin B deficiency. In the complete absence of zinc, reproduction is seriously affected. In addition to the prostate gland, zinc is concentrated in the human body mostly in the liver and spleen, although the pancreas contains considerable amounts. Diabetics know that the insulin they take is generally "protomine zinc insulin." The necessity of zinc in the pancreas can best be explained from the point of view of the diabetic. (See diabetes questions and answers section). In relation to the person suffering from diseased prostate gland much of the same applies. The sick prostate gland contains far less zinc than the normal one. According to one group of investigators, concentrations of zinc in the normal prostate tissue and in the swollen gland are about the same. But cancer of the prostate and infection of the prostate result in considerably less zinc in the gland. Others have found that the zinc content of the prostate is lowered in any disorder of the gland. So it seems that zinc may be just as important to the functioning of this gland as it is to the pancreas. Sperm is richer in zinc than any human tissue studied, yet the testes are relatively poor in this element. From this observation alone, it would seem that zinc is related to spermatic physiology. It is conceivable that the prostate acts as nothing more than a purveyor and receptacle for zinc until ejaculation occurs and at this time zinc is incorporated in the sperm in a perhaps essential capacity. Certainly, under the conditions of the experiments, the unfailing appearance of Zn65 (that is radioactive zinc) in prostatic fluid suggests that prostatic fluid without zinc would no longer be prostatic fluid.

All foods related to good nutrition seem to contain some elements of zinc, but particularly rich in zinc are onions, brown rice, whole eggs, oatmeal, cocoa, molasses, chicken, peas, beans, mussels and wheat germ, oysters, beef liver and gelatin.

### BIBLIOGRAPHY

Bourne, Geoffrey, *Biochemistry and Physiology of Nutrition,* Academic Press.

Bragg, Paul, *Building Powerful Nerve Force,* Health Service Co.

Lake, Thomas T., *Treatment of the Prostate By Physical and Manipulative Therapy,* Health Research Pub.

Rodale, J. I. and Staff, *Encyclopedia of Common Diseases,* Rodale Books, Inc.

# VARICOSE VEINS

**Question:** How is the disease phlebitis related to varicose veins and what exactly is going on in the body housing these conditions?

**Answer:** Phlebitis is a condition of inflammation of the veins, involving blood clots. Varicose veins are veins which have become deformed and twisted. It follows that deep phlebitis should be looked for whenever there are varicose veins, however mild or early. If a person has varicosities there is most often evidence of phlebitis in the deep veins, meaning the veins deep in the muscles of the legs rather than on the outside where they can be easily seen. The veins deep inside the leg muscles are designed to carry about 80 percent to 90 percent of the return flow of blood from the feet. If something goes wrong, so that one of these veins is plugged, the veins on the outside of the leg near the skin surface must take over. In the effort to cope with the additional work, these veins dilate, twist and do their best to empty the blood from feet and legs. They enlarge and the valves which control the blood flow cease to function properly. The veins which join the deep set of vessels to the exterior ones become filled with blood and big varicose veins spray out over the ankles. If a doctor injects or cuts or strips away these ugly veins on the outside of the leg, he is removing the only possible channel for the blood to flow through, since the deeper veins are already plugged. So the patient may end up far worse off than before the operation. If vitamin E is used instead of an operation it can produce collateral circulation about the obstructed deep veins by calling into play the unused networks of veins lying in wait for emergency utilization. We have such venous reserves just as we have reserves of brain, lung and liver. Alpha tocopherol (vitamin E) mobilizes them, and more. It has the unique power of enabling tissues to utilize oxygen better and hence, the devitalized and congested leg tissues of the phlebitic are receiving the equivalent of more oxygen. One other solid suggestion for the prevention of varicose veins and phlebitis, apart from taking E, and making sure your diet is well chosen, is proper exercise. Some of our present day difficulties with the blood vessels of our feet and legs come from the fact that we just don't use them enough. We need exercise, every day. Walking is one of the best and cheapest forms of exercise. Walk in the country, if you can; walk barefoot, if you can; walk before breakfast and before lunch and before dinner, if you can. But regardless of how much you can walk, do plan your day's activities, no matter how much trouble it takes, to include at least one good walk every day. You'll be amazed at how thoroughly the exercise will get the blood to flowing through in your feet and legs. When you rest, put your feet up on something—a footstool if you're sitting, a pile of cushions or the arm of a chair if you're lying down.

**Question:** I've heard that constipation has a definite relationship to varicose veins. Is that true?

**Answer:** It is believed that a cause of varicose veins is constipation. And this is in relation to the fact that the greater incidence of varicose veins occurs on the left side of the body. The vein leading out of the left side of the testicle opens into the renal vein at right angles without a valve, while the right vein opens into the main vein obliquely, with a valve. The way the left vein leads into the main abdominal vein results in a greater pressure on that side. On the left side of the abdomen is the part of the colon which descends to the rectum. It crosses directly over the left spermatic vein. On the right side is the ascending colon which does not cross over the right ascending spermatic vein. This is the circumstance which could well hold the secret of varicose veins. The removal today of so much of the fiber from foodstuffs often leads to delay in the passage of the colonic contents and to an increase in their weight. Since a relatively low pressure can arrest the blood-flow in even the largest veins, a loaded iliac colon (the left side) can easily obstruct the left spermatic vein and induce a varicocele. In the standing or sitting position, the entire weight of the contents of the ascending colon, which are fluid, is transmitted down to the cecum (area where small intestine opens into the colon). If the colon is overloaded, pressure will be considerable—more, perhaps than the pressure exerted on the other side by the contents of the descending colon. This may explain why plain, everyday varicose veins are not much more common on the left side than on the right—a little more common, but not much. Very serious varicose veins, the kind that confine one to bed, are many more times common on the left side. Lying down in bed results in far less pressure by that part of the colon on the right side of the body, but there is still plenty of pressure on the left side where the colon, overloaded, lies over the large vein that goes to the legs. Even though the structural parts of an individual's anatomy can account for varicose veins appearing, it would not be the case with the absence of the primary cause—that is, constipation. Without that these structural differences would not produce any disease at all.

**Question:** Can a person be born with varicose veins?

**Answer:** Varicose veins is not believed to be a congenital state. One reason can be based on a look at percentages. Congenital malformations in general affect not more than 5 percent of the population whereas varicose veins afflict (20) times this many people. Also, malformations with which one is born are caused by an error in the fusion or joining together of certain parts in the unborn child; they are not errors in mechanical conception, as varicose veins are.

Asking the question of a person being born with varicose veins brings up a point concerning medical opinions generally favoring the notion that man is the only animal subject to varicose veins, because he is the only one that walks upright. And his troubles with the veins in his legs began when he assumed his upright position. How does it happen then, that nature could have made such a grievous error in the anatomy of man? Allowing him to assume an upright position many, many years ago and not in some way adapting him to this position so that he could no longer suffer from it? We see that varicose veins are not only confined to people above the reproductive age whose physical efficiency may be considered unimportant to the human race. The disorder has been found in healthy young persons as well. Such a tremendous incidence of varicose veins is evolutionarily quite incompatible with the view that the veins are a structural weak link—a failure in man's evolution. The struggle for existence has never been so kind as to permit a state of affairs like this.

## BIBLIOGRAPHY

Bragg, Paul, *Building Powerful Nerve Force,* Health Service Co.

Bronson, Barnard Sawyer, *Nutrition and Food Chemistry,* J. Wiley and Sons.

Davis, Adelle, *Let's Get Well,* Harcourt, Brace and World.

Fraser, Harris, D., *The Man Who Discovered The Circulation of Blood.*

Poynter, C. W. M., *Congenital Anomalies of the Arteries and Veins,* University of Nebraska Press.

Rodale, J. I. and Staff, *Encyclopedia of Common Diseases,* Rodale Books, Inc.

# BACK TROUBLE

**Question:** What are some of the causes of backache?

**Answer:** Backache, the common terminology for "low back pain," can be brought on by various physical ailments. But before going into a listing of these ailments you should know that the kind of backache most common and most easily prevented is the one that is a result of poor posture, improper furniture or the wrong kind of movements in daily life.

Otherwise, backache is often attributed to arthritis, unusual muscle strain, a recent or long-forgotten bump, or a wrench occurring especially during periods of fatigue. It may indicate a slipped vertical disc, an infection of the urinary or genital tract, an acute illness, general ill health, a local infection somewhere in the body or even overweight. We are surprised at how often physicians will indicate that backache may be psychosomatic, meaning that the ache is a physical symptom of some strong emotional strain or frustration.

**Question:** I often wake up in the morning with a mild backache. I have just passed thirty-five and am wondering if the backache is just one more indication of middle age catching up with me or what?

**Answer:** If you specifically get up in the morning with a backache take a good look at that bed you are putting yourself to rest on every night. It's probably too soft. All you've got to do is watch a person who is lying in a hammock and you will get an exaggerated idea of what a soft bed does to one's body. If you lie on your back, your chest is constricted. If you lie on your stomach, the spine and hips are extended into a completely unnatural curve. Therefore your bed should be firm and flat. In most cases, modern mattresses and springs tend to "give" too much which is why many people find it better to sleep with a fairly thick board between the mattress and springs so that the bed does not curve beneath your weight, no matter how you sleep. This kind of bed board can be bought or you can make it yourself from a piece of plywood.

**Question:** Does body type have anything to do with susceptibility to backache?

**Answer:** Tall, thin people are inclined to be more susceptible
to backache from poor posture than are short, stocky ones. Obviously the muscles that support the back have a bigger job to do—
more actual back structure to support and a longer distance over
which the support must be given. In the pregnant woman or the
woman who has had children, the muscles that support the abdomen are weakened, the abdomen sags, pulling on the back to
deepen the curve there and produce a full-fledged case of "swayback." This can be easily corrected if caught soon enough. If not,
backache is a likely result. And teenagers who grow too fast tend
to slouch so that their height will not be noticed. Rounded shoulders are the result.

**Question:** I've accepted the fact that poor posture contributes
to my occasional "low back" discomfort. Everyone tells me to
'stand up straight.' What does that often-used phrase mean in
terms of my doing something specific to improve my posture and
prevent backache?

**Answer:** Stand in front of a long mirror after your next shower
and look at your posture. You should be able to hang a straight
plumbline from your ear to the ball of your foot and half of you,
perfectly balanced, should be on each side of the line. You can
strengthen and improve the tone of the stomach muscles by lying
flat on the floor and raising up to a sitting position without using
hands or arms. Or you can lie flat and lift one leg after the other
in the air, slowly. If you want something even more simple to aid
in that "stand up straight" look, try exercising your abdominal
muscles while you go about your own business. Pull up and in on
them, tucking your buttocks beneath you. Hold your head high,
your chin in and your shoulders up. When you lift something
heavy, bend your knees, get close to the object, and when you lift,
let your legs do the work rather than your back. When you bend
don't bend at the waist with your knees straight. Bend your legs
and keep your trunk straight.

Remember that the entire basis for proper posture is the fact
that the spinal column is designed to stand in a straight line, with

segmented curvatures to provide flexibility and absorb stress from the base of the skull to the pelvis.

## BIBLIOGRAPHY

Alsakar M.D., Rasmus, *Conquering Colds and Sinus Infections*, Groton Press

Bragg, Paul, *Building Powerful Nerve Force,* Health Science Pub.

Davis, Adelle, *Vitality Through Planned Nutrition*, Macmillan Co.

Shepard, John Frederick, *The Circulation and Sleep*, Macmillan Co.

Warmbrand, Max, *The Encyclopedia of Natural Health,* Groton Press.

# ARTHRITIS AND RHEUMATIC DISORDER

**Question:** What is the difference between arthritis and rheumatism?

**Answer:** The meaning of both words and their relationship to each other should be made clear at the very beginning. Arthritis is a disease of the joints and it is considered one member of the "rheumatic" family. Rheumatism includes disorders such as lumbago, neuritis and sciatica which involve the muscles and nerves as well. Rheumatism is the heading of a category of diseases which includes forms of arthritis. We must bear in mind that all arthritic and rheumatic diseases arise as a result of the same or similar health-deteriorating influences and can only be corrected through sound systemic care applied in conformity with sound natural healing principles. This approach is applicable in all cases of arthritis, those that develop slowly and insidiously as well as those that set in abruptly and that are accompanied by high fever or sudden intense pains. We must never forget that the factors that have made this disease flare up suddenly have most often been laying the foundation for its eruption for a long time.

**Question:** I know that arthritis is a disease of the joints and that in various stages and forms it affects millions of people in this country. What are the early symptoms of this disease?

**Answer:** As a rule arthritis develops slowly. It can take years until one is aware of the serious manifestations. Even when the onset seems immediate, with severe pain and high fever, you must realize that the elements that have given rise to it have been operating for a long period of time.

Pain or discomfort in the joints or limitations of motion—even very temporary—should serve as signals warning that arthritis may be in the making and that attention is required. The disease in its earlier stages is often mild, and immediately cared for can be readily overcome. Unfortunately, initial symptoms are often so superficial that only rarely are they recognized as the beginning of arthritis. A feeling of numbness or stiffness, creaking and cracking of the joints, occasional twinges, cold, clammy hands and feet —these are some of the early symptoms of the disease. In most cases these early warnings are either completely ignored or treated in an off-hand manner, for such routine procedure only contributes to the more severe forms of the disease. An aching back may suddenly clear up and not recur for a long time; it is therefore easily forgotten. Yet such experience, especially when recurrent, should serve as a warning that you are courting ill health. Numbness of the joints or stinging sensations are not always sufficiently annoying, yet, if not taken care of, can lead to more serious things. A burning sensation of the feet or twinges, as well as a feeling as if ants were crawling under the skin, should all serve as warnings that something is wrong. Do not overlook care when these early symptoms exhibit themselves.

**Question:** What exactly is going on in an arthritic joint as compared to a healthy one?

**Answer:** Looking at a joint reveals several interesting points. The adjoining ends of the bones are covered by a semi-soft elastic tissue called the cartilage, which cushions the joints and minimizes friction and strain. The inner surface of the joint cavity is lined with a membrane, known as the synovial membrane, which secretes a light, yellowish semi-liquid fluid that keeps the joint lubricated. The ligaments and muscles hold the joint together and in place.

In health the bones are well-knit and firm, and the circulation of the blood and lymph, which carries food and oxygen to the tissues and picks up waste materials for elimination, is unimpeded. The cartilages are pliable and serve to protect the joints against undue friction or strain. The synovial membrane secretes the fluid that is necessary to keep the joints lubricated. The muscles and ligaments possess the tonicity and springiness for firmness and balance.

In arthritis, many changes affecting the function and structure of these tissues take place. The joints become large and swollen, or shrivel up and waste away. The bones become either thickened or wasted and the adjoining surfaces often present irregular, rough, or jagged appearances. The circulation of the blood and of the lymph is impaired and this deprives the tissues of nutrition and oxygen, and interferes with the elimination of the waste materials. The cartilages lose their pliability and become brittle and dry. The function of the synovial membrane becomes damaged, causing either an excess or a lessening of the secretions. As the disease progresses the membrane becomes completely worn out and the secretion dries up completely. The ligaments and muscles lose their tone and their flexibility, wasting away or becoming congested and thickened. All these destructive changes do not develop at once. An impairment in circulation, with an inflammatory condition of the synovial membrane or the cartilages, is usually the change that manifests itself in the earlier stages of the disease. It is only as arthritis progresses that the more advanced destructive changes develop and the more severe manifestations of the disease become apparent.

**Question:** How does arthritis begin to develop in one's body?

**Answer:** Arthritis is a disease that often strikes because of a disturbance in body metabolism, or arises as a result of prolonged abuse or abnormal wear and tear of the joints. It develops also as an aftermath of injury or trauma. Earlier acute illnesses when improperly treated often plant the seed for this disease in children as well as adults. The presence of abscessed teeth and tonsils, and similar "focal" or "local" infections may precede the onset of this crippling disease. A sudden injury such as a fall, a sprain, a fracture, or lacertation, or any infectious disease when neglected or treated the wrong way, can leave a defect which later develops into arthritis. Frequently, a shock to the nerves, tension over a prolonged period of time, arteriosclerotic changes in the body, all set up chain reactions that ultimately form different types of arthritis.

**Question:** Why does arthritis persist? If we can locate the problem why isn't it solved easily and effectively for most people?

**Answer:** When those casual, prearthritic symptoms become annoying, they are usually passed over or more often supplemented with a remedy prescribed to provide relief. Bicarbonate of soda to neutralize acidity, codeine to relieve pain, the barbiturates or bromides to check nervous symptoms—these are some of the typical remedies used. These drugs may help to relieve distressing symptoms or lessen discomfort, but since they accomplish this by means of sedation or stimulation and since they do not eliminate causative factors, they have no corrective value and fail to overcome existing systemic disturbances. It is deplorable that most sufferers fail to recognize the futility of these conventional remedies, so far as permanent correction is concerned. Very seldom are they aware of the temporary nature of these remedies, and seldom do they recognize the need for more fundamental changes. Cathartics induce bowel action, but do not overcome intestinal sluggishness; in fact they only increase the intestinal weakness. So-called alkalizers may relieve digestive upsets, but as long as the causes of the "acid" condition remain, the symptoms will recur, with ever greater damage as the ultimate result. Barbiturates or bromides may quiet nervous symptoms, but in time cause greater impairment to the nervous system, and are responsible for many breakdowns. A stimulating drug or physiotherapy may temporarily improve the circulation and provide relief, but unless fundamental corrective measures are employed, the underlying disturbances are not overcome and the diseased condition continues to grow worse. These or similar remedies may mask or modify symptoms, but they fail to promote the needed correction and ultimately cause more disease.

**Question:** Please tell me about drugs and their effects on relieving and subsequently curing the pains of arthritis.

**Answer:** It seems that a month doesn't go by without publicity given to a new "miracle" drug being found that will cure arthritis. But it has been shown over and over, one such drug does not perform any sort of miracle cure for this crippling and devastating disease. As for the more established drugs, it also holds true that the old, conventional remedies may provide that needed relief, but the experiences of sufferers of this disease have amply proved their ineffectiveness as far as permanent benefit is concerned. These preparations may actually add to the damage.

Now we will look at a treatment breakdown, giving the more commonly discussed drugs, conventional and new, and beginning with the "miracle" drugs that have recently gained the spotlight.

**Sub-Question:** What are the "miracle" drugs that have received all this criticism?

**Answer:** The sulfa drugs have been introduced as remedies against what is commonly identified as "infection." The theory explaining the action of the sulfa drugs is that they counteract or destroy infection by choking off the supply of oxygen to the bacteria. Still it is known that the sulfa drugs can cause great damage to the body. Diseases of the blood, injury to the kidneys and liver, nervous disorders, impairment to the heart and skin diseases are only a few of the many aftereffects that often follow their use. These remedies often inactivate the acute processes of the so-called "infection" or suppress some of the symptoms of disease, but they neither overcome the lowered resistance nor eliminate the toxic condition that exists. Also the antibiotics such as penicillin, streptomycin, aureomycin and chloromycetin have been proved to be powerful bacterial poisons. As such they may be effective in checking or modifying certain disease symptoms of their manifestations. However, since disease does not originate in germs but in bodily perversions or metabolic disturbances, the mere modification or suppression of the symptoms of disease or their manifestations without the eradication of the underlying abnormal bodily conditions will fail to bring about basic systemic correction. Cortisone and ACTH are two more of the outmoded "wonder" drugs that have been used on arthritis sufferers. Cortisone is a substance derived from the adrenal glands, which have a lot to do with maintaining resistance to disease. ACTH is a substance made from the pituitary or master gland of the body. They are interrelated because when ACTH is injected, it stimulates the adrenal glands to produce cortisone. When cortisone was first tried out on arthritis patients results were astonishing. Pain disappeared, a sense of well-being and a good appetite returned. However, it was soon admitted that improvement stopped as soon as treatment stopped, so cortisone was no cure. In addition, it was found that, in many cases, extremely serious aftereffects ensued. Patients might be disturbed mentally. They might develop abnormally round faces and abnormal growths of hair. ACTH might bring about diabetes or high blood pressure. Then, too, any slight infection becomes a menace to the patient taking these drugs, for he is not aware of the infection. If it should be tuberculosis or something equally serious, it can develop into a fatal disease rapidly, while the patient, delighted that he feels so well, overexerts himself and courts disaster. No one knows exactly how these side effects come about, but we do know that glands are powerful influences, governing all the activities of the body. Taking a hormone, any hormone, is bound to disturb the delicate balance among the glands and bring abnormalities. Cortisone and ACTH, as well as other drugs affecting glands, should never be taken except under strictest supervision, so that the side effects can be detected early.

**Sub-Question:** What of aspirin and its effects?

**Answer:** Known technically as acetylsalicylic acid—aspirin—is a coal-tar derivative and belongs to the salicylate group of drugs. It is regarded as a remedy "par excellence," and is so extensively used in treatment of arthritis that it often becomes a habit and a routine. There is no question that aspirin may provide relief, but often the user must pay a very grave price, physically and emotionally. The continuous use of aspirin, over a long period of time, can be quite harmful. Long, consistent salicylate therapy may depress the production rate of immune bodies in the organism. And it is of considerable importance to recognize that evidence of the persistent activity of the rheumatic infection may be masked by the continuous use of aspirin, which abolished temporary symptoms and signs including fever. Thus, the aspirin is converting an active rheumatic condition into a chronic state. And is a patient benefiting when his ailment is converted from its acute state to a chronic one? Also, the possibilities of aspirin in large dosages causing poisoning in the system cannot be overlooked. Intoxication can result in profuse sweating, cold extremities—either with or without a fall in body temperature, rapid or irregular pulse and occasionally albumin in the urine. This toxic effect of aspirin can be a severe irritant to the stomach lining, can cause internal bleeding or hemorrhages, for it destroys vitamin K, which aids in the coagulation of the blood, and it may bring serious trouble to patients susceptible to coronary thrombosis.

**Sub-question:** What of the drug cinchophen and its effects?

**Answer:** Cinchophen is prescribed to promote the excretion of uric acid from the system. Nevertheless it is an extremely dangerous drug that can cause great harm. Why this is still used is somewhat of a mystery. Cinchophen, apparently, disturbs the skin, the digestive tract, the heart, the kidneys and the liver. Sometimes the degeneration of the liver occurs so extensively that repair cannot be effected. Also, hepatitis and jaundice are known to set in. Although the excretion of uric acid through the kidneys is important in fighting arthritis, this drug's use is just too dangerous. Most unfortunate is that the toxic effects of cinchophen may come on suddenly with so much injury to vital structures that nothing can be done to save life.

**Sub-Question:** What of codeine and its effects?

**Answer:** Codeine is obtained from opium, resembles morphine, and contains many of the toxic properties of these drugs. It is used in many conditions for which opium is usually administered and although it is less efficient than morphine it has the advantage of being less constipating and less liable to habit formation. Symptoms of poisoning by it have been vascular excitement, exhilaration, then depression with great anxiety, nausea and vomiting; pale, cool, clammy skin, slight contraction of pupil and sleeplessness with slight delirium. Codeine is often prescribed to relieve the excruciating pains of this disease. It is, however, regarded as having no therapeutic value and its use only leads to more enervation with an increase of toxemia and damage.

**Sub-Question:** What of actual vaccines and their effects?

**Answer:** The principle behind the administration of vaccines as treatment is that the vaccines would stimulate the production of antibodies to combat or destroy invading bacteria. Vaccines that are used are either freshly prepared from the patient's own secretions or are stock vaccines put up ready for use. This form of treatment has proven to be a failure. Its application is often followed by dangerous consequences. Vaccines are supposed to aid in building up the immunity of the body, yet advocates of this practice concede that they do not know how they work and can never be certain of obtaining results. While the aim is to increase immunity, it is admitted that the effect may frequently be the very opposite. It is recognized that relief of pain following the use of vaccines often results from the fact that the reactive powers of the body have become impaired or depressed. But this certainly does not mean increased immunity. When the suppressive effect wears off, greater sensitivity with increased suffering often follows. When we think we are building immunity we may actually be suppressing the reactive powers of the body, and when this desensitization wears off it may be followed by greater sensitivity and more pain. So far as the psychological effect of vaccine therapy is concerned, it is interesting to note an experiment in which the injection of a plain salt solution and small doses of aspirin for patients suffering from osteoarthritis resulted in improvement in 86 percent of the cases. It is known that any form of treatment that raises the hopes of the patient has a profound psychological effect and makes the patient feel better. This, however, is not of lasting value.*

**Question:** I have a friend who suffers the pains of arthritis in both hands. She has been visiting a health spa in Arizona in the past year for therapy. Is this a reasonable way to treat arthritis?

**Answer:** Sufferers from arthritis frequently visit spas or bathing resorts or travel to distant places in the hope that mineral baths or a change of climate, will, in some miraculous manner, promote their recovery. If you accept that this form of treatment derives benefits of only a temporary nature, you can look at the positive aspects of the mineral baths which make them, to some degree, worth taking. Apparently minerals are absorbed through the skin and there is sulphur present in the minerals. We know that sulphur is important for the efficient working of the human body. It is present in every plant and animal cell. In the body, the muscles contain about half the sulphur, while bones and skin contain most of the rest. Foods high in protein are also high in sulphur, for it is contained in several of the amino acids or forms of protein which are absolutely essential to human welfare. It is possible that the arthritic patient may be lacking in sulphur and that the mineral bath helps to make up this deficiency. It was found, particularly, that the cystine content of the fingernails of arthritic patients is far lower than that of normal subjects. Cystine is one of the forms of protein which contains a lot of sulphur. It has also been found that the cystine content of the fingernails increased after a sulphur bath. In summing up, we do not object to a visit to the spas. Any change that takes the patient away from the monotony or stress or strain of his daily existence is a psychological plus and a benefit.

---

*The Encyclopedia of Natural Health by Max Warmbrand, N.D. D.O.

However, it is essential that we realize that such a change is not sufficient to restore health. Diet, exercise, occupational therapy are the areas to concentrate on for permanent improvement. The mineral baths and the relaxing effects from a change of climate are undoubtedly helpful, but the benefits are only of a temporary nature, unless the sufferer also recognizes the necessity of a complete reformation in his mode of living.

**Question:** Can you give me a rundown of good nutrition, including foods and vitamins, and its role in the treatment of arthritis?

**Answer:** We believe that arthritis can be prevented and that its severity can be greatly lessened by following the proper diet. The pathway to arthritic disease is lined with desserts, candy, soft drinks, heaping spoons of sugar in coffee or tea, jelly and white bread. The surest preventive is fruits and vegetables, a diet in which refined carbohydrates are completely absent and vitamins and minerals are provided in abundance by natural food supplements.

Most sufferers from arthritis eat similar diets. Usually they consist of high amounts of carbohydrates, low trace mineral intake and low consumption of foods rich in vitamin B. The large amount of white sugar ingested displaces, by its large calorie count, an equal amount of calories from foods that contain the elements the body needs. Sugar is the surest means of knocking the calcium-phosphorus balance out of kilter. It always boosts the calcium count while lowering the phosphorus: then, when the effect has worn off the reverse occurs, with the phosphorus shooting up and the calcium becoming depressed. The elimination of sugar, along with white flour and alcohol, both of which have a similar effect, is the most important step in the cure of arthritis. That alone should put the arthritic on the road to cure, but further insurance lies in abandoning completely the use of refined and processed foods. These foods seem to contain many elements which adversely affect the calcium-phosphorus ratio in the blood. Can intelligent diet be such an impossible assignment that arthritis victims would rather suffer the crippling pain than change their bad food habits!

**Sub-Question:** What in the way of proteins should be used in my diet?

**Answer:** Protein foods provide the building materials of the body and are essential for adequate nutrition. However, the types of protein used by the sufferer from this disease are of extreme importance. The heavy, concentrated proteins create a great deal of uric acid and other poisonous by-products, which are harmful in this disease. The arthritic must make certain that he obtains proteins from foods that are easily digestible and produce a minimum of toxic by-products. A great deal of confusion exists with regard to the protein foods. Many are under the impression that meat, fish and eggs are the only foods that supply the right kind of protein. This is a grave mistake. It is known that millions of people in different parts of the world live on very little meat or no meat at all; and yet, how vigorous and sturdy most of them are compared to us. They obtain their protein from dairy products, the lowly potato, nuts, grains, and the green leafy vegetables and fruits. The vegetables and fruits actually do provide a rich, incomplete protein in easily digestible form, although in much smaller quantities than more concentrated protein foods. All foods contain protein: there are none without it. The question is merely which of them provide the more valuable protein. For the sufferer from arthritis it is without question that the more easily digestible and less concentrated proteins obtainable from vegetables, fruits, the potato, and soft, nonfermented cheeses are the ones to be recommended.

**Sub-Question:** What of eggs and milk. Are a quantity of those foods reasonable for my diet?

**Answer:** Eggs are considered a valuable source of protein and yet they are regarded as partially harmful in the diet of the arthritic. Eggs are not easily digested, owing to their rich fat content. In addition they contain a relatively large amount of a wax-like substance known as cholesterol, which when not properly disposed of contributes to the formation of gravel and stones, and leads to hardening of the blood vessels. Since our need is to dissolve deposits and soften hardened tissues, and since the metabolic functions in this disease are definitely impaired and may therefore be unable to adequately utilize and/or dispose of cholesterol, the use of eggs is inadvisable. Milk and milk products are a good source of complete protein, and for that reason are favored. The use of such mild, soft cheeses as cottage cheese, pot cheese, farmer's cheese, or the Italian bland cheese known as ricotta is generally healthy. However, since all concentrated protein foods are sources of uric acid, only moderate quantities of these cheeses should be used, and in the early stages of arthritic treatment it may be advisable to restrict their use or omit them altogether. Milk, too, should be used sparingly, or even be eliminated in the early stages of the treatment. Allergists are aware of the fact that in cases of allergy, milk is not always a suitable food. Since allergy is regarded as a factor in many cases of arthritis, it is not wise to use a food that may prove detrimental.

**Sub-Question:** Grains are essential foods, but are they beneficial to the arthritic sufferer's diet?

**Answer:** We know that bread is supposed to be "the staff of life." However, grains are concentrated starch foods and acidforming. Thus they are difficult to digest and cause an excessive amount of lactic acid fermentation which is a detriment to health. If used at all grains should be used but sparingly, and then only in the whole, unrefined form. White flour products should be completely omitted. The whole grains are highly recommended for their rich mineral and vitamin content. However, there is no need to depend on them for our minerals and vitamins, for these valuable elements are available in great abundance in raw vegetables and fruits, which lack the detrimental effects of the grains.

**Sub-Question:** I know that vitamins in proper dosage are necessary for a healthy body, but I have heard that too much vitamin D in the treatment of arthritis can be harmful. Is that true?

**Answer:** Vitamin D in massive doses had gained great popularity as a form of treatment of arthritis, but the bad aftereffects that began to manifest themselves following its use considerably cooled the ardor with which it was originally advocated. Too much concentrated vitamin D is known to harden numerous body tissues until they are much like stone. Vitamin D causes extensive calcification. In arthritis, the need is not to promote mere increased or decreased calcification but to bring about an improvement in general metabolism with restoration of a more normal calcium metabolism. When this is brought about, correction will take place and the calcification or decalcification that may be indicated will take place, to the extent that it is possible. So, obtain the needed vitamin D from natural sources and not in the form of concentrates. Fruits, berries and green leafy vegetables and exposure, moderately, to the rays of the sun are all ways of acquiring the vitamin D supply.

**Question:** I have heard that going without solid food for a period of time could help in controlling arthritis. Could you explain this further?

**Answer:** Going without food—or fasting—can help the body to rebuild the reserves that have already been wasted and is a step in the direction of renewed health. Fasting conserves the bodily reserves and lessens the strain placed upon the digestive organs. The arthritis sufferer must not overtax his digestive system by eating too much food or the wrong kind of food, and he must be careful not to combine foods improperly. The arthritis sufferer must rebuild his wasted energies, and when he abstains from food completely for a few days, or follows a more restricted dietary program, his digestive organs are given a chance to rest. Abstinence from foods helps the body to dispose of toxins that have accumulated, and also provides rest to tired and overworked organs. A short fast, two or three days, can be very valuable. This "cooling off" period helps detoxify the body, rest the digestive organs and promote increased elimination of toxins by way of the kidneys, the intestines and various other channels of elimination. There is a recommendation for a beginning fast by following a limited diet. Devote a day or two to liquids only. Take grapefruit juice or hot vegetable broth only about every two hours, or if this is too strenuous, adopt a fresh fruit diet, for two or three days, taking one kind of raw fruit at a time about every two or three hours or whenever hungry. If you wish to do it at a slower pace, use the fresh fruit in the morning and all through the day, eating an evening meal composed of a large raw vegetable salad, baked potato, and one steamed vegetable. Your system will then gradually become adjusted to controlled fasting. For arthritis victims this only helps hasten the relief of pain.

**Question:** Please tell me something about water therapy and its effects on arthritis.

**Answer:** Aside from the spas and health resorts we reviewed earlier, there is the at-home, everyday use of water and bathing that can be of great comfort to arthritis sufferers. The hot bath promotes more rapid skin elimination and encourages increased kidney function. This helps rid the body of the toxic wastes that have clogged up the internal mechanism of the body; it improves the circulation and provides great relief of pain. Comfortable hot baths, to which two glassfuls of epsom salt are added, are most beneficial. These baths should be taken at first daily; but then may be reduced to one every second day. The baths are best taken before retiring since in most instances they relax the body and induce sound sleep. To maintain the bath at an even temperature, the hot water should be kept dripping into the tub while the bath is taken. Following the hot bath, the arthritis sufferer should, without drying, immediately get into a robe and then retire. He should make certain to be well covered, and if this induces sweating, he should not let this worry him for this is helpful. The "secret" here is that in causing perspiration, toxins are being eliminated by the way of the skin, and more active kidney elimination is induced. Hot epsom salt baths can be used with great benefit in most cases of arthritis. Of course, there would be some cases where this treatment would be too stimulating and tend to keep a person awake. The bathing habit should, of course, be regulated to correspond to the individual's wants and needs.

**Question:** What about the use of cleansing enemas. Can they be habit forming?

**Answer:** A warm, cleansing enema has many benefits for the arthritis sufferer and it is not habit forming. The enema promotes the elimination of stagnant accumulations from the colon, relieves flatulence, improves the abdominal circulation by removing obstructing wastes and helps to break up congestion. It also reduces the strain on the heart as well as on the other internal organs of the body such as the liver, the gallbladder, the pancreas and the lungs. Use warm cleansing enemas with care and only when they are actually needed. When used too often they tend to wash away the natural secretions, and cause needless irritation to the inner lining of the colon. They have to be used very cautiously in cases of spastic or sensitive colon and should be completely avoided in acute appendicitis or other acute intestinal inflammations such as ulcerative colitis, ileitis and diverticulitis. Many people shy away from the enema altogether, yet resort to laxatives or cathartics which are not only habit-forming but actually weaken the intestinal tract. The enema neither rebuilds nor strengthens the colon. It merely removes the accumulated residue and should be considered a temporary expedient until the necessary corrective measurs have strengthened the colon and restored normal intestinal functioning.

**Question:** I've always associated gout, in a humorous way, with Benjamin Franklin and his big toe. Recently, I've heard that this condition is to be taken seriously; that it is a form of arthritis and it causes much pain. Can you tell me more about this disease?

**Answer:** The big toe story has a basis in truth, for when this disease strikes the big toe usually suffers most, but other joints are also affected. Gout is a defect in the body's chemistry. There is an increase of uric acid in the system and this is caused not merely by wrong food or too much food, but by a defect in the body metabolism. Gouty arthritis, in its advanced stages, is the result of a toxic irritation set up around the joints by crystals—uric acid crystals—and an inflammation in these crystals brings on the attack of gout. The kidneys can secrete only a certain amount of the uric acid crystals that accumulate in the body. The rest is accumulated in the tissues, and when they deposit in the points, gouty arthritis ultimately develops. The crystals accumulate and may appear around any joint, but usually, around the big toe and also on the external ear, cartilages, the bones, and the tendons. The deposits themselves are painless. But joint inflammation is painful, and the inflammation arises because the joints are trying to get rid of the "foreign" substance that does not belong there. Furthermore, the kidneys may be damaged and uric acid kidney stones may form. Gout is caused by wrong or high living. Overindulgence in unnatural foods and alcohol may bring on an acute attack or hasten the development of crystal accumulations. Overweight makes the disease more severe and more difficult to control. Richly concentrated acid-producing foods, as well as highly processed and refined foods and beverages, may cause a defect in metabolism and lead to the accumulation of uric acid crystals. Sufferers from gout or gouty arthritis must plan a complete change in their foods and dietary habits in order to ultimately overcome the tendency to produce and accumulate excessive amount of uric acid in the system and help to eradicate the disease. Sufferers should avoid anchovies, clams, fish roe, scallops, shrimp. Also they should omit brains, duck, goose, liver, pork, sausage, tongue. Gravies, meat soups, meat extracts, alcohol and cola drinks must be excluded. Sugars, cake, pastry, ice cream, sharp spices and condiments are also taboo. These foods and beverages cause an increase in uric acid and therefore must be eliminated.

**Question:** How do I apply exercises—calisthenics—to my everyday routine to help combat arthritis?

**Answer:** Exercise is totally helpful and many arthritis sufferers are discovering that deep body massage and a well-planned program of physical exercises, as well as various manipulative techniques can be a great aid to them. When applied correctly these manual types of care improve circulation, loosen up rigid and stiffened joints and do much to relieve pain and discomfort. As proper exercise increases the size and number of blood vessels, new routes for the delivery of more oxygen develop. This is a vital factor in the health of the arthritis sufferer. Deep breathing exercises, for one, provide a deep sense of well-being as they develop better chest muscles, strengthen the abdominal muscles and highly invigorate the whole system. Deep breathing exercises are most effective when done slowly, rhythmically. If it is inconvenient to lie down, do them before an open window. But be sure that you inhale and exhale slowly, deeply, rhythmically, as the key to success here is to take in fresh, pure oxygen and dispose of carbonic acid gas. All the cells of the body need oxygen and the joints of the arthritis sufferer are starved for it. The arthritis sufferer needs oxygen which is carried by the blood to the small hidden pocket sites where pain and crippling is often pronounced. The best thing to do in order to compile an effective, detailed exercise program would be to consult with your physician and see what progressive, positive movements would be most beneficial. The areas that you do want to cover include: the stiff neck, upper and lower back, hip joints, stiff feet, the legs, the wrists, the hands and general good posture— standing up straight. Perhaps, as a beginning we will recommend stretching and rotating exercises for arthritis sufferers. In doing stretching exercises, lock your hands behind your head, then slowly stretch them upward, against resistance while rising slowly on your toes. Stretch and keep stretching as this is wonderful for the whole bodily function. In doing rotating exercises, stand up straight, place hands on hips and rotate your body slowly, first to one side then to the other side. Rotate as far as possible and try repeating this five times.

Once your program is selected it is necessary to be aware of the right way to do your exercises. Exercises should be done slowly and rhythmically and should be carried through the full range of motion. Don't let pain dissuade you from working out, although discontinue exercises temporarily when pain becomes acute. But don't forget to get back to them as soon as the acute pains lessen. Some pain is to be expected, since your joints and muscles have become stiff and rigid and are now being stirred up and reawakened. And for greatest benefit, when you do these exercises daily, make sure that your body is warm and relaxed. Physical exercises when carefully applied are of great help in arthritis, but they are merely part of a complete health-rebuilding program. A carefully planned diet, an abundance of rest and sleep, the comfortable hot epsom salt baths, emotional control and peace of mind are essential parts of the overall health-building program and must be followed if the arthritis sufferer is to get well.

**Question:** Is sleep an important factor to the arthritis sufferer and are there specific things he should know about rest and relaxation as well as turning in for the evening?

**Answer:** Pains and stiffening of the joints put the arthritis sufferer's body under much internal tension. This tension drains vitality and aggravates the arthritis condition. Sleep and rest are essential if the circulatory system, the hormonal system, and the various vital organs of the body such as the heart, lungs, the kidneys and the liver are to regain the necessary self-regenerative powers. Maintaining a balance between activities and rest is necessary if one is to get well. Rest helps to overcome inflammation as the joints need sufficient rest. For example, a "localized rest" is provided when pressure and strain is kept off the inflamed joint or through the use of temporary support, while an abundance of sleep and complete body rest helps to rebuild the health and strength of the whole body. During rest and sleep, the body promotes its own drainage of congested fluids and helps to eliminate toxic waste products. This is especially the case when rest and sleep are part of an overall health-building program. When a joint is severely inflamed, enforced exercises have to be suspended until the acute inflammation has either been overcome or is in the process of being broken up. During the period of rest, the body's organs regain their strength and are enabled to carry out the various detoxifying processes that help to get the arthritis sufferer well. Rest helps to rebuild the functions of the colon, the kidneys, the liver, and the other organs of elimination and this helps rid the body of accumulated toxic waste products. You store up energy with lots of sleep and even if you feel the need for 12, 14, or 16 hours sleep a day, don't fight it. You never sleep too much when your body needs rebuilding and strengthening.

Many arthritis sufferers pay for inside and outside tensions with sleeplessness. These tensions interfere with sound sleep. Insomnia can be overcome by adopting certain natural practices which induce a normal desire for sleep. First, have your evening meal early, and keep it light. A light meal is easier for a tense stomach to digest. Always remember when sleeping and resting to choose the most comfortable position. If the arthritis sufferer does not have sufficient freedom of movement (this takes in size of bed consideration) to alternately relax different sets of muscles he awakens feeling cramped and tired. Try to relax yourself toward evening. Perhaps a pleasant book, soft music, even simple meditation will ease tension and lead the way to sleep. Often a short walk will relax this tightness of feeling. Try a hot epsom salt bath before retiring and if this should prove too stimulating for a full night's sleep try the bath in the morning before a short rest period instead. And make sure your feet are warm in bed by using, when necessary, either a hot water bottle or a heating pad. Cold feet interfere with sound sleep. It will be a blessing if you can train yourself to float into pleasurable nothingness. It will induce relaxation and make you more contented and cheerful. It will help you digest your food, and will hasten quick recovery. Make the sleep habit a lifetime habit.

**Question:** How does rheumatic fever develop? There have been a few cases of it recently in the grade school that my young son attends and I'm really not too sure what it is all about.

**Answer:** Rheumatic fever is a disease that most often affects the young. About 75 percent of all who suffer from rheumatic fever are below the age of 20. Rheumatic fever was originally regarded as an acute rheumatic disease of the joints. However, since many of these cases are followed by heart damage, many authorities now classify it as a disease of the heart. The disease often affects other parts of the body as well. The kidneys, the nerves, as well as many other parts of the body. When the nerves are affected, it gives rise to the condition known as chorea. Malnutrition or poor dietary factors, fatigue, poor environment, or any of the influences that lower the resistance of the body, play an important role in the development of this disease. The reason we have a preponderance of rheumatic fever among the poor is simply because these unfavorable factors predominate in the homes of the poor. In discussing a well-balanced diet it should be pointed out children contracting rheumatic fever seemed, in general, to eat a small supply of eggs. Having a proper supply of natural fatty substances in the blood seems to correspond to rheumatic fever being at a minimum. The substance in egg yolk that gives protection is some kind of fatty substance although researchers are not sure what that is—can it be lecithin or something else?—that protects against rheumatic tendencies. There is positive evidence of the relationship between adequacy of diet and susceptibility to this disease. A well-balanced diet plus wholesome living conditions will not only help toward rapid recovery but will protect the heart against damage as well.

**Question:** What of the importance of good posture in the prevention of rheumatism?

**Answer:** Good posture is essential for good health, and it is particularly important in any disorder in which bones, joints and muscles are involved, for these are the parts of the body which suffer most from bad posture. Good posture can work wonders, even though there are some postural handicaps that cannot be overcome without the aid of professional therapy. But perfect posture, in general, is so simple that there can be no disagreement as to what it means. It means keeping one's body in balance so that there is as little strain as possible on muscles, bones and nerves, when one stands, walks, sits or works.

Many people suffer from sad off-balance posture as they slump over and stick out their stomach unattractively. The best thing to do to begin correcting bad posture is to pull in on the muscles of the stomach. In doing this the curve in the back would straighten out, which in turn would correct a flat chest and rounded shoulders. As these fall into place the legs and feet would assume their rightful positions. Good posture would be the result, with the head, shoulders, knees and feet in perfect alignment with pelvic structure —that is, the bony base to which one's legs are attached and which contains the abdominal organs. A plumb line dropped from one's ear to his ankle would be straight and would divide him in half, that is, half of his body weight would be found to be on each side of the line. Actually, the only hard thing about regaining good posture is reminding yourself of it. Once the muscles have been strengthened, you'll have good posture without giving it another thought. But meanwhile, make a habit of studying your reflection in shop windows when you're walking on the street. One glance will remind you to pull in those stomach muscles. At home or at work decide on some one object—a calendar, a window, a piece of furniture that will be your constant reminder, every time you look at it, to correct your posture. You may be saving yourself years of agonizing pain with arthritis later on in life.

## BIBLIOGRAPHY

Aschner M.D., Bernard, *Arthritis Can Be Cured*, Arc Books, Inc.

Bourne, Aleck William, *Health of the Future*, Penguin Books.

Bourne, Geoffrey, *Biochemistry & Physiology of Nutrition*, Academic Press.

Broadstreet, Hobart, *Spine Motion*, The Provoker Press.

Cooper, Francis Lenna, *Nutrition in Health and Disease*, Lippincott.

Davis, Adelle, *Let's Eat Right to Keep Fit*, Signet Books.

DeFrost, Clinton Jaris, *Arthritis and Folk Medicine,* Holt, Rinehart & Winston.

Sure, Barnett, *The Vitamins in Health and Disease,* Williams & Wilkins Company.

Warmbrand, Max, *How Thousands Of My Arthritis Patients Regained Their Health,* Arc Books, Inc.

# THE HEART AND HEART DISEASE

**Question:** I have heard the heart referred to as a "living pump." Could you tell me more about its movement and function in relation to that descriptive phrase?

**Answer:** In order to fully understand the action of the heart as the "living pump" which it is, it would first be necessary to take a look at what the heart is pumping—which is, the blood. Today, the importance of the blood and its effect upon our health and well-being is fully recognized, and it is now well known that any impairment in its composition or functioning will vitally affect the whole body. The blood is a vast world of countless microscopic entities known as the blood cells. This enormous population confined within the blood vessels lives and functions in a sea of fluid known as the plasma. About half our blood is composed of plasma, while the other half is made up of the blood cells that live and work in it. There are two types of blood cells, the red and the white. The red pick up the oxygen in the lungs and carry it to all the cells of the body, while the white fight off "infection" or foreign matter. Each cubic millimeter of blood in the average healthy human body contains about five million red cells and between 7,500 and 10,000 white cells. Since the average adult body contains about six to eight quarts of blood, we can readily visualize that the number of red and white blood cells living and working within the confines of our body reaches astronomical figures. The blood vessels are airtight to prevent air from coming in contact with the blood. In case of injury, the blood of a healthy person clots quickly when coming in contact with the air and this seals the wound. The blood contains such clotting substances as thrombin, prothrombin, thromboplastin, ionized calcium, and fibrinogen, which make it clot whenever it comes in contact with air. In case of injury this protects us against hemorrhage. When some of these elements are not present in the blood in adequate amounts or when an imbalance exists, the blood may not be able to clot properly, and in case of injury we would be in danger of bleeding to death. On the other hand, under certain conditions the blood may tend

to clot too quickly, and then we are in danger of blood clot formation. This is the condition that exists when clots form in the heart,
the brain or the extremities. In the healthy body the clotting mechanism is in perfect balance and the problem of too rapid or incomplete clotting of the blood arises only when our health has become
impaired sufficiently to upset this balance.

Now that we have taken a look at the blood and its makeup
and functions, we are ready to examine the heart as "living pump."
Physically, the heart is a hollow organ about the size of a fist.
The inner part of the heart is divided into four chambers, two on
the right and two on the left side. The upper chambers are separated from the lower chambers by a partition, each side of which
contains a valve that opens downward. These valves open when
the heart muscles relax, and close when contraction sets in, thus
regulating the flow of blood to the body and to the lungs. This
process continues without a stop throughout life. Each side of the
heart is completely separate from the other and handles its own
particular part of the circulation. Thus, the heart may be regarded
as a dual pump, taking care of two separate but interrelated cir-
culations. The right side of the heart pumps the poison-laden
and oxygen-deficient blood brought back from all over the body
into the lungs, where carbon dioxide is given off and new oxygen
is taken in. The left side of the heart receives the purified and
oxygen-enriched blood from the lungs and then pumps it into the
general circulation for distribution to all parts of the body. The
heart has no piston *per se* but, like a pumping engine, keeps steadily pumping, contracting and relaxing its muscular tissue at regular, rhythmic intervals, forcing the flow of blood ever onward and
forward.

**Sub-Question:** Can you give me a step-by-step description of
how the heart performs?

**Answer:** When the poison-laden and oxygen-depleted blood is
brought back to the heart, it is first emptied into the upper right
chamber. From there it is pumped into the lower right chamber,
and then carried by two blood vessels (the pulmonic arteries) into
the lungs. After giving up its carbon dioxide and taking on a new
supply of oxygen, it is then carried through an entirely different
set of blood vessels, this time four in number, two from each lung,

into the left upper chamber of the heart. From there it is pumped into the lower left chamber and then pumped into the general circulation for distribution to all parts of the body. The upper chambers of the heart fill with blood during their moment of relaxation and empty their content into the lower chambers during their moment of contraction, both sides performing their work simultaneously. This work goes on continuously, each pumping beat of the heart, each "lub-dub" taking about nine-tenths of a second or about 72 times per minute. While the heart maintains its work continuously, it also has a period of rest. It rests after each beat, and each interval of rest is about twice as long as the beat itself. The total volume of blood in our body is six to eight quarts. Since three ounces of blood pass through the heart with each beat and since each beat of the heart takes about nine-tenths of a second, the total volume of blood passes through the heart and completes its cycle throughout the body in about one to one and a half minutes. The lower chambers of the heart also work in teamlike fashion. They fill during their momentary state of expansion, and force the blood onward during their moment of contraction. It is important to bear in mind that while each side of the heart handles its own specific part of the circulation, both sides do work in unison. Both upper chambers of the heart fill with blood during their momentary state of expansion and empty their contents into the lower chambers during their moment of contraction.

**Sub-Question:** Is the intensity with which the heart works pretty much fixed or is it determined to an extent by the demand placed upon it?

**Answer:** Rapidity or intensity with which the heart works is determined to a great extent by the demand placed upon it. When the heart has less work to do, it is more at ease and usually works at a slower pace. When a greater demand is made, it is forced to work at a faster pace and with greater intensity. When an organ is called upon to do more work, it must be supplied with more oxygen, and the heart must pump more blood to supply it. When we run or exercise, more oxygen is needed and the heart is forced to pump harder. The same is true when we eat. To digest food, the digestive organs require more oxygen, and the heart is called upon to do more work. More oxygen is required during illness, and this again increases the work of the heart. The same holds true in excitement, tension, overwork, or any type of emotional stress. When the heart is in a healthy condition it possesses a great deal of power and strength that provide not only for the regular demands of the body, but also a great deal of reserve power to meet unforeseen or unexpected needs. Whenever a demand for an increase in circulation arises anywhere in the body, this demand is transmitted with lightning speed to the pumping mechanism of the heart and when the heart is in good health, it unfailingly responds to this need. Whenever the heart is called upon to spend its reserve powers recklessly, it will ultimately become worn out, and its efficiency and power will become impaired. Reserve powers should be handled and channeled carefully, so that they may be at our disposal during periods of actual stress, as in the case of disease, accident or shock, and it is the height of folly to squander them carelessly, thereby jeopardizing our health and our life. Even this powerful organ, the heart, with its amazing recuperative powers, can ultimately become weakened and worn out and that, to protect ourselves against this possibility, our reserve powers must not be needlessly drawn upon.

**Question:** What are the interrelated functions of the arteries, capillaries and veins and what are their associations to the heart?

**Answer:** The work of the heart is to pump the blood and keep it in circulation. The work of the arteries is to carry the blood with the oxygen and other nutrient materials to every cell of the body. The arteries are made up of soft, elastic muscle fibers and are strong enough to take the entire impact of the pumping heart. They expand to receive the blood that the heart pumps into them and contract to force it onward. Since the arteries are made up of living tissue they also require food and oxygen, but as in the case of the heart, they obtain their nutrients not from the blood that flows through them, but from the blood brought to them by their own special arteries, known as the vaso vasorum. An intricate system of nerves plays an important part in regulating their functions. Starting with the main artery, the aorta, which emerges from the lower left chamber of the heart, the arterial system branches into a vast network of large and small arteries, reaching out in every direction and carrying blood with its oxygen and other nutrient elements to every cell and part of the body. The large arteries sub-divide first into smaller arteries, then into still smaller arteries, and finally into the minute, hairlike blood vessels known as the capillaries. The actual interchange between the blood and the tissue cells takes place not in the larger arteries or their smaller subdivisions, but in their smallest subdivisions, the capillaries. The capillaries are the minute, thin-walled hairlike channels stretching many thousands of miles, that reach into every nook and corner of the body, that transport food and oxygen to all cells of the body and remove their waste products. This interchange between the capillaries and the tissue cells takes place through the very thin walls of the capillaries and proceeds at billions of dif-ferent points simultaneously. The capillaries, the smallest sub-division of the arteries, also form the beginning of the veins. Neigh-boring capillaries merge and form small veins—venules—out of which by fusion the larger veins are formed.

The veins carry the oxygen-depleted and poison-laden blood back to the right side of the heart to be pumped into the lungs for purification and re-oxygenation. This is done while the arteries carry the oxygen-enriched blood to the cells. However, even though both types of blood vessels are part of the same circulatory system, they nevertheless show certain structural differences. The arteries, closer to the pumping heart and exposed to its full force, have a much heavier load to carry and because of this are more powerfully developed and possess a greater resiliency than the veins. The veins, though, possess a unique feature not found in the arteries. They are covered with valves to prevent the blood from flowing back. The veins, being farther away from the heart and not bene-fiting to the same degree as the arteries from its pumping force or "push," need this added protection.

**Question:** I know that heart disease is the greatest single killer in this country and that the statistics seem to be growing year after year. But what is it that people are specifically talking about when they discuss disease of the heart?

**Answer:** This good question needs to be answered with great detail for heart disease, that is most common and takes the greatest toll of human life, is to be grouped into three categories: hyper-tensive, coronary or arteriosclerotic, and valvular or rheumatic.

It is important to discuss these in depth. Too often the layman speaks of heart attack in so very loose terms not knowing the inside workings of heart disease and how attack (and sickness) is brought on.

**Sub-Question:** What exactly is hypertensive heart disease?

**Answer:** Hypertensive heart disease is the type that develops as a result of or in connection with high blood pressure. When the blood pressure is high, the heart is forced to work harder to maintain the circulation. In order to cope with this added demand, the muscle of the heart is forced to enlarge. While an enlargement of the heart is a characteristic sign in this type of heart disease, it should be remembered that a mere enlargement in the size of the heart is not in itself an indication of heart disease. Athletes or physically active persons often develop large heart muscles as a result of their physical activities. However, a muscle that becomes larger because of normal physical exertion is a healthy muscle, while a muscle forced to enlarge when too much work is thrust upon it is sapped of its strength and ultimately becomes worn out and damaged.

Hardening of the arteries (arteriosclerosis) is the most common form of this particular division. And the hardening is the factor that most often contributes to the development of high blood pressure. This, of course, does not preclude high blood pressure being affected possibly by nervous tension, glandular disorders, certain types of kidney disease, and a change in the volume or consistency of the blood. The arteries in the healthy individual are soft and pliable and are able to expand and contract effectively. When the arteries become hard and brittle and the inner walls thicken and narrow, they are unable to do their work efficiently, and the heart is forced to pump much harder to maintain circulation. Hardening of the arteries occurs in two forms. One, the pipestem or calcifying type, caused by the gradual deposit of calcium within the walls of the arteries. The other, the cholesterol type of hardening, develops when cholesterol, a chemical substance of fatty origin, is deposited within the walls of the arteries. This second type is most often the case, wherein the cholesterol thickens the artery walls, reducing the amount of space in the arteries for the blood to circulate. If this happens in the big arteries that feed blood into the heart, it creates an impediment to its flow, and if it occurs during an emergency or severe activity, when the blood need increases, it will bring about heart symptoms such as chest pressure pains and an angina attack. Cholesterol is a compound which is a constituent of gallstones. In reasonable amounts it is needed by the body. It is an important part of the nerve tissue. It also opposes those elements which destroy red blood corpuscles. It is the substance that reduces wateriness of cells, giving them a semi-solid character. It has other important functions, but when it increases too much, accumulates in places where it has no business to be, it can be a great hindrance to the proper circulation of the blood. Cholesterol is found only in animal fats, not in vegetable fats. Our prosperity is causing us to live off the "fat" of the land so to speak, the fat is clogging up our arteries and the result is deaths from heart attacks. Therefore, animal fats should be on the low side in the diet. We can be fairly liberal with vegetable fats, especially corn, soybean, sunflower and fish oils, for these are noted for their ability to reduce the cholesterol in the blood.

Now we should take a closer look at exactly what is meant by blood pressure. This is the pressure exerted within the blood vessels by the circulating blood. The blood pressure is measured to determine the amount of pressure that exists in the arteries when the heart is at rest. The pressure when the heart is at rest is known as the diastolic; the pressure when the heart is in action is known as the systolic. While both pressures are important, the diastolic is the more important as an index of normality since it indicates the degree of tension or strain existing in the circulatory system. The blood pressure fluctuates in accordance with the influences that affect the body as a whole. The same influences that affect the heart also affect the blood pressure. While blood pressure tends to rise with age, this is not to be regarded as a normal condition. It occurs because as people grow older their blood vessels tend to lose some of their elasticity. This, however, need not happen since the blood vessels can be kept resilient, thus maintaining the blood pressure of the younger age range, even as the person grows older. In the healthy person, the inner lining of the arteries is smooth and flexible, and the blood can flow through them easily. But when calcium or the fatlike substance, cholesterol, is deposited on the walls of the arteries, the arteries become hard and brittle, and the channel through which the blood flows becomes narrower. This slows down the circulation of the blood and in time may cause the formation of a clot which will obstruct the circulation completely. When a clot forms in one of the arteries of the heart, we have what is known as a coronary thrombosis or coronary occlusion. In this condition, the affected part of the heart is deprived of its circulation and failing to get its nourishment and oxygen, ceases to function. This is commonly known as a heart attack. When the circulation to the kidneys becomes affected, their functions become seriously impaired. They are unable to eliminate the toxins effectively and the fluid balance in the body becomes upset. This in turn overtaxes the arteries and the heart and leads to their breakdown.

**Sub-Question:** What exactly is coronary or arteriosclerotic heart disease?

**Answer:** While hypertensive heart disease arises from a general hardening of the arteries or high blood pressure, coronary or arteriosclerotic heart disease develops from a hardening of the coronary arteries, the arteries that supply the heart with its blood supply. Coronary or arteriosclerotic heart disease begins with hardening of the coronary arteiries. When the coronary arteries become hardened, the condition is known as coronary sclerosis. When the condition develops, the heart is unable to receive an adequate supply of oxygen and other essential nutritious elements and ultimately begins to break down. Since this condition usually develops slowly and insidiously, the early stages are often not easily recognizable. However, as the disease progresses, certain warning symptoms or disturbances often begin to show up. Among these are heaviness or pressure on the chest or excruciating pains in which the chest feels as if it were tightly clamped in a vise, squeezing all life and strength from it. During these attacks the pains often radiate into the left shoulder, sometimes into the right shoulder, occasionally into the abdomen. These attacks, known as angina pectoris, occur when one of the coronary arteries is in a spasm because of an insufficient supply of oxygen. It is fortunate that these attacks last only for a short time, usually no more than a few seconds, sometimes one or two minutes, rarely more than 10 or 15 minutes.

Where they continue for more than a half hour, a coronary thrombosis must be seriously suspected.

**Sub-Question:** What exactly is valvular or rheumatic heart disease?

**Answer:** Valvular or rheumatic heart disease is another type of heart ailment that takes a terrific toll of human life. In it, the valves of the heart have become thickened and scarred and are unable to close or open completely. As a result, some of the blood leaks through or is pushed backward. This disrupts the normal circulation and places a great strain upon the heart. To cope with this condition, the heart is forced to enlarge and because of the added strain it ultimately becomes worn out. Fortunately, a great deal of repair is possible in many cases. Proper care strengthens the heart and promotes the necessary readjustments which enable it to function better in spite of the damage. The damage in valvular or rheumatic heart disease can be readily discerned, as a physical examination will disclose the presence of an enlarged heart, but cannot always easily be recognized. This is because the presence of an enlarged heart does not necessarily indicate a heart that is tired or hardened or scarred as well. In other words, even though the heart appears normal it is actually unable to maintain an efficient circulation. This should be kept in mind, for many persons assume that once they have had their periodic health check-up and have been told that their heart is in good condition, that they have nothing to be concerned about. But close attention, particularly in advanced cases, can reveal the damage and worn-out condition. Changes such as a wasting or shrinking of the heart muscle, advanced stages of fatty degeneration, or infiltration of fatty deposits in the heart muscle fibers are more easily recognized, and many abnormal symptoms such as difficult breathing, night asthma, rapid or slow pulse, swelling of the liver, fluid in the abdomen and chest, help one to make a correct diagnosis. Be alert to the fact that mild disturbances such as dizziness, blurred vision, or digestive distress often arise from minor heart damage. In some cases, several such areas of minor damage become confluent and cause a major defect, leading to so-called sudden death. While the sudden death in these cases is due to a major organic breakdown, it is really the outgrowth of a slow form of deterioration that has reached its peak. One of the conditions often found in the later stages of heart disease is known as heart block. The function of the heart is supposed to be one of perfect balance, maintaining a rhythm by the nervous system and a special control in the heart muscles, the sinus rhythm. When this special control becomes impaired, an imbalance between the upper and lower chambers of the heart develops. While the upper chambers function at a normal range, the lower chambers are unable to keep in step. In reality, no breakdown limits itself exclusively to one side of the heart. Failure in most cases begins with the left side but usually will affect the right side as well. When the left side of the heart is unable to pump the blood it receives from the lungs, the lungs cannot empty any more blood into it, and as a result there is a backing up to the right side of the heart. The engorgement that results produces a stretching or dilating of the heart, and causes trouble.

**Question:** Is the hardening of the arteries a condition to be considered inevitable?

**Answer:** First, it is interesting to note that the number of cases of heart and circulatory disease has increased to a great extent not in the older population but in the younger age groups or those in the prime of their lives. While age, of course, is relentless, hardening of the arteries does not run the same course. It is not considered an inevitable process of aging and this thinking has been confirmed by many leading authorities in the heart disease field. What should be emphasized to all people, despite their particular age groupings, is a healthy heart goes hand in hand with moderation in diet, exercise, and the drive under which people work, as precautions to be taken.

**Question:** Where do vitamins B and C fit in regarding cholesterol in the diet and its relationship to the hardening of the arteries?

**Answer:** We know that cholesterol is found in large quantities in the fatty foods of animal origin such as eggs, milk, butter, cream as well as the fatty meats and fish. Therefore, it seems logical to assume that by controlling the intake of these foods, hardening of the arteries could be eliminated or greatly lessened. However, many of our authorities were not satisfied by this assumption. Although they were aware that a restriction in the intake of cholesterol-rich foods benefited their patients, they were still confronted by questions that seemed most puzzling. For one thing, they noticed that many persons who consumed large quantities of the cholesterol-rich foods did not suffer from hardening of the arteries; for another, further research disclosed that not all types of cholesterol, but only a special type, giant cell cholesterol, caused damage. Finally, they began to realize that hardening of the arteries does not develop merely from an intake of cholesterol-rich foods, but from a faulty utilization of them. And it is this—the faulty utilization of them—that pertains to vitamins B and C.

Vitamin C is an important factor in keeping down the cholesterol in the blood. Also C plays a strong role, directly or indirectly, in the curing of heart disease generally. This vitamin maintains the blood vessels and connective tissues in good condition, preserving the strength of the capillary walls. And this one function of vitamin C is of great importance in considering the underlying causes of heart disease. There are many parts of the vitamin B complex that have been shown by medical research to be of value in the prevention and cure of hardening of the arteries. Included in this group are choline, pyridoxine, inositol, and thiamin. Choline is a lipotropic agent, which means that it combines readily with fats or oils, and thus hastens the removal of fat deposits. Pyridoxine is also involved in the process by which the body uses fat. It is believed a deficiency of pyridoxine can cause high blood pressure. And when people think they are getting enough of this daily they are mistaken. About half the pyridoxine in grain is lost when the grain is processed. The processing of milk and meat, cooking and stewing food result in substantial losses of the vitamin. Any amount of heat or light damages pyridoxine. Regarding inositol, research has proven that the daily taking of the vitamin inositol will result in lowering of the cholesterol content of the blood, having to do with the metabolism of fat. White sugar, ice cream, soft drinks, cereals rob our body of thiamin and if you are a heart case this robbery is extremely dangerous. Thiamin deficiency impairs the function of the heart, increases the tendency to extravascular fluid collections and can result in terminal cardiac standstill. Therefore, we can see that if we assure ourselves sufficient vitamin B, preferably in the form of supplements to the regular diet, such as brewer's yeast, desiccated liver, wheat germ and blackstrap molasses, we will be moving in the right direction toward preventing undue accumulation of fatty deposits in the artery walls.

**Question:** I've heard that it is vitamin E, in particular, that has been causing much talk about prevention and cure of heart disease. Why is vitamin E placed in such a position?

**Answer:** Vitamin E oxygenates the tissues and also has anti-bloodclotting ability. This is so very important to prevent death through thrombosis or a blood clot. In the case of thrombosis, the taking of sufficient vitamin E can save lives, by preventing blood from forming clots. Research has shown the undeniable truth about vitamin E's multifaceted, heroic role in the body's metabolism, particularly in the heart muscle itself and in the circulatory system of every human being and every animal thus far studied. Vitamin E is oil-soluble and is found in the oils of wheat germ and many other plant seeds. It is also present to some degree in leafy vegetables and other plants. It is found in varying amounts in animal tissues (including man's), generally being concentrated in fatty tissues and in organs such as the heart and the liver. Vitamin E is a vital component of the blood as well. Milk and eggs also contain the vitamin. Vitamin E is composed of seven forms of what chemists term "tocopherols." They are labeled alpha, beta, gamma, delta, epsilon, eta and zeta—but alpha is the only form which has been shown to be very active in the animal or human body. Although the other tocopherols may someday be found to play a role in metabolism, as yet alpha tocopherol alone is synonymous with vitamin E in the minds of most present-day researchers. Henceforth, when we use the term vitamin E, we are referring to alpha tocopherol, not to the other inactive forms of the vitamin.

Many researchers have established that vitamin E is an anti-oxidant and an oxygen-conservator. These properties signify that vitamin E possesses the ability to improve the cell's function and prolong its life. As an anti-oxidant, vitamin E delays the oxidative process which turns cells "rancid," and it prevents oxygen from combining with other substances to form the deadly hydrogen peroxide which hastens the death of a cell. This fact has been proven on human beings, on animals, and on tissues which have been removed from recently-killed animals. As a natural anti-oxidant and oxygen-conservator, vitamin E affords the body many advantages. First, when richly supplied with vitamin E, the cells of the body are able to perform more efficiently—not demanding as much oxygen for metabolic processes, thereby freeing more oxygen for those cells and organs needing it. An ailing heart for example, not demanding as much oxygen as before—that is, before the therapeutic dose of vitamin E—does not have to pump as hard to convey blood to the cells. Its work is considerably lessened, consequently easing the strain—an extremely important factor in heart ailments. Also, the heart muscle itself is more richly nourished with oxygen through its main source of blood supply, the coronary arteries. These two factors, less work and more oxygen, partially explain why the vitamin has a direct, beneficial, seemingly miraculous effect on lagging hearts, and on normal hearts as well. Researchers have stated that vitamin E therapy is equivalent to being placed in an oxygen tent—without the inconvenience, of course. But equally important as its oxygen-hoarding properties is the fact that vitamin E "guides" the oxygen in proper functions. When cells have a scarcity of vitamin E, they tend to release their oxygen, which then combines with the cellular wastes to form poisons dangerous to the cells. Also vitamin E is a vasodilator: it opens arteries so that more blood can flow through the circulatory system. This is of particular significance to victims of circulatory disorders such as hardening of the arteries. Still another recognized property of the amazing vitamin E is its ability to maintain normal permeability of cellular membranes, notably the capillaries. If the capillary walls become too impermeable, their function of feeding the cells is impaired; on the other hand, if the walls become too permeable, they leak out their precious cargo into the extra-cellular spaces where it does not belong, and, thus, the cells are deprived of nutrition. So we see that a constant supply of the proper substances is needed to sustain the tricky equilibrium maintained between the capillaries and the cells. Along with other substances such as vitamin C, vitamin E maintains the normal integrity of these walls, preventing them from becoming too permeable or impermeable, or from breaking.*

---

*Vitamin E, Your Key To a Healthy Heart* by Herbert Bailey.

Although no one is certain of the exact chemical process involved, there is ample evidence that vitamin E is closely related to healthy muscles. And let's not forget that the heart is the most important muscle!

**Question:** Explain to me about body metabolism and its relationship to the heart and heart disease.

**Answer:** Scientists have now begun to realize that diseases of both the heart and circulation arise from an impairment in the metabolism of the body. The term metabolism covers a wide field. It embraces all the known and unknown functions of the body and all the known and unknown chemical and physiological processes that break down our food and oxygen so that they can be utilized by the cells. The digestion and assimilation of food, the secretion of the endocrine glands, the functions of the nervous system, the elimination of toxins, and the thousand and one chemical and physiologic changes that take place continuously within our organism are part of this complexity. Anything that impairs these functions leads to a derangement in nutrition, affects the elimination of toxins, impairs glandular functions and causes a chemical imbalance. These are the impairments that exist and are part and parcel of our so-called metabolic diseases. Diabetes, arthritis, diseases of the kidney and the liver, the various nervous disorders, as well as the diseases of the heart and blood vessels, all belong to this category. The changes that take place in heart disease also develop when the body attempts to cope with conditions or influences that threaten life; as such, they are part of our defense mechanism. When the heart has more work to do than it can safely handle, its muscle is forced to enlarge. This change allows the heart to cope with the increased amount of work and to protect it against collapse. When the blood vessels become thickened and hardened or when scar tissue develops in the muscle or in and around the valves of the heart, these changes too arise from an attempt to repair an inflamed or damaged area, and to prevent the damage from spreading. The ability of the body to seek to maintain its metabolism and in the case of the heart to make these repairs, even though they bring with them an alteration in structure, is instrumental in saving human life.

**Question:** We hear so much talk about blood pressure—high blood pressure and its factor in causing heart disease. What I don't know too much about is low blood pressure. Can you fill me in on this and tell me if it is a great concern to people with heart trouble?

**Answer:** While high blood pressure is of greatest concern, it is well to know that low blood pressure too must not be neglected since this also may be a warning that our health is not in the best condition. Low blood pressure may result from extreme debility, weakened arteries, a bad heart, an impoverished blood supply, poor quality of the blood, or a disorder of the glandular system. While it is not well known, a stroke or coronary thrombosis or other abnormal clotting phenomenon may develop in cases of low blood pressure, and may result from a weakened heart or a poor circulatory condition.

It is interesting to note that low blood pressure is not considered, in general, a cause, but an effect that could result from heart disease. The viewpoint of the medical profession towards low blood pressure—if it is not connected with specific disease—is rather tame. In some cases of below-normal blood pressure the cause seems to be exceptionally elastic arteries and this is a good thing. It can indicate the expectation of a longer life as with the low pressure the hardening of the arteries will be slow to develop. Other viewpoints tell us that low blood pressure may be simply an indication of poor nutrition and it is often accompanied by low blood sugar, low basal metabolism, anemia or hyperthyroidism. In general, low blood pressure seems to go with people who do less of everything than other people do. That is they may not eat enough or exercise enough which causes their glands to slow down and decrease their secretions. In cases of outright starvation, of course, the blood pressure is always low. In direct regard to heart disease, if we are talking about causes, it is the high blood pressure that one has to be most concerned about.

**Question:** What role do the kidneys play in heart disease?

**Answer:** The function of our kidneys plays a vital role in the development of high blood pressure as well as heart disease. The type of kidney disease that contributes to the development of these diseases is known as glomerular nephritis. The glomeruli are the filters of the kidneys. Each kidney contains billions of these microscopic filters whose job it is to filter out the fluids and expel the waste products from the body. When the kidneys become impaired, they are unable to function efficiently, and as a result, many of the toxins are retained in the system and the fluid balance in the body becomes disrupted. This places an added strain on the heart and raises the blood pressure. Stress or strain, or excessive wear and tear, caused by overwork or the accumulation of toxins or substances of an irritating nature that are generated within the system as a result of improper functioning or are taken into the system with improper food and drink or in the form of drugs or chemicals, cause disorders in metabolism that ultimately manifest themselves in one or other of our metabolic diseases, which include the diseases of the heart and blood vessels.

**Question:** I know that obesity is alien to a healthy heart, to a totally healthy body, for that matter. Could you relate the specifics of overweight to heart disease?

**Answer:** It has been proven conclusively that excess weight is not only dangerous to the heart and the vascular system, but also to all the other vital organs of the body. It is from every conceivable standpoint a menace to health. Excess weight is considered more dangerous in the 35 to 45 than in the 45 to 54 age groups. This is clearly in line with the greater increase in mortality from heart and vascular disease in these age groups, and undoubtedly one of the factors responsible. Hardening of the arteries and high blood pressure, percentage-wise, seem to be much more of a problem to overweight and obese individuals than to those of normal, proper body weight. Other disorders which seem to find comfort in obesity include: diabetes after 40; gallbladder disease, and degenerative arthritis.

Many persons realize that excess weight is harmful but lack the will to control appetite, and therefore keep looking for short cuts. Many doctors will still prescribe thyroid extracts, which often cause great harm, and others prescribe other hormones or laxatives of various kinds; it is well known that none of these remedies accomplishes its objectives. Clear and simple, to be a heart case and to be overweight is to be shamefully negligent. And the most important factor in losing weight is to eat less. Begin by cutting food intake in half, and eating very little or none of the food you crave most. Discontinue white bread, white cereals, cakes, cookies, candy, creams and all kinds of sauces. Use more of raw and stewed fruits and raw and steamed vegetables along with a small quantity of your favorite protein, once daily. Exclude all sugars and all fat foods. Discard the use of condiments and spices. Table salt tends to put weight on by retaining fluid in the system and should therefore be eliminated from the diet. Furthermore, do not be afraid to go without a meal or two. An eliminative regimen for a day or two, or even several days at a time, will work wonders . It will hasten the reducing process and benefit you immensely. You should not only think of reducing weight, but also of rebuilding the body, at the same time, to the point where the glands and the digestive organs function normally. After the correct weight is established, this program of living must be continued if you are to maintain your gain. A heart case should consume a low-fat diet. It is important to reduce the total amount of fat in the diet of a person with a heart condition, but in making the decision as to which types of fat to retain in the diet, bear in mind that the egg is a whole food, out of which a living thing will emerge. It has the germ of life in it if it is a fertile egg. There just isn't any comparison with milk and dairy products. The egg is far superior from every point of view, besides containing a large quantity of lecithin which is the antidote to the cholesterol that the egg contains. Don't eliminate fats altogether. This can lead to depression. Fat is necessary for the proper absorption of carotene which is the first step in the body's manufacture of vitamin A. As for the meal program for the day, skipping breakfast is not desirable as a means of losing weight. The consensus is that you will be so hungry that you will eat more the rest of the day. All in all, reduction in daily calories adds years to your life. This is especially important to a heart case because the heart is overtaxed in helping to digest heavy meals. Cut down on the amount of food you eat and eliminate entirely fried foods, coffee or tea or maté, soups, bread and flour, dairy products, sugar and salt. And remember, vitamins should be taken with meals because they aid the digestion. By aiding the digestion, the vitamins seem to break down or homogenize the fats so they are not stored as fat. This is of major significance in a reducing program.

**Question:** Can you give me a general nutrition breakdown as it regards the treatment of diseases of the heart and blood vessels?

**Answer:** That's a big area to cover, particularly since nutrition pertaining to heart and blood vessels cross-cuts into good nutrition for vital organs in general and the whole bodily function as well. But there are a few specifics we can talk about here. First, we can say that fat foods should be excluded, although the benefits of lecithin in eggs, an animal fat, are thought to make them beneficial enough to combat the cholesterol. Then there is table salt, which should be excluded in heart disease, hardening of the arteries and high blood pressure, because sodium, one of the elements of table salt, is eliminated through the kidneys and can be a burden to them. Also the intake of too much protein can prove unhealthy to people with heart problems. And not getting enough lecithin in the diet can cause trouble, as lecithin is known to counterbalance the cholesterol in the body. Unfortunately, so many of our processed foods retain the cholesterol, but destroy the lecithin in the hydrogenation process. This is common, for example, in hydrogenated fats which are the shortenings used in pastry and for frying. Lecithin is so very important, and it is made in the liver, provided certain ingredients are present there. We might say then, why not manufacture it ourselves? Well, one of the B vitamins, choline, and the unsaturated fatty acids (sometimes called vitamin F) must be present for the liver to make lecithin. And unfortunately, we have done our best to remove both these substances from our national diet, so the supply of lecithin suffers. Be sure then to get lecithin in your diet from such natural sources as seeds (melon seed, sunflower seeds, cereal seeds etc), cold-pressed oils and food supplements.

**Sub-Question:** What of tobacco and alcohol and their effects on the heart?

**Answer:** Let's take tobacco—smoking—first. No one has to be told that smoking is harmful. While recent reports in the press have dealt primarily with the effect of smoking on the lungs, its detrimental effects on the heart, although not as exclusively publicized, have been known for a long time. A person who has heart disease is committing slow suicide if he is a smoker—whether it be of cigarettes, cigars or a pipe. Something in tobacco prevents the heart from functioning properly. And there is so much clinical evidence of this that it should convince even the most skeptical. The following information will give you some known facts regarding tobacco and its harmful nature regarding blood vessels, capillaries, etc. Cigarette smoking is known to cause a definite constriction of the blood vessels, it raises the blood pressure and the pulse rate, being extremely detrimental to persons who are susceptible to cardiac trouble. Also we know that vitamin C is able to reduce the cholesterol in the bloodstream. And it is now known that smoking reduces the supply of the body's vitamin C. We begin to see the vicious circle forming. If smoking reduces the supply of the body's vitamin C, one can see the danger to a heart case—smoking would tend to cause an increase in the cholesterol content of the blood. It is also known that smoking disturbs the fat metabolism and raises the fat level of the blood to a point where it becomes a contributing factor in the development of heart disease. The development of giant particles of fatty materials has been found in the blood of constant smokers. Regarding alcohol, we can begin by saying that it destroys vitamin B in the body. Also, it damages the nervous system and the brain. It affects the liver, many of the glands, destroys red corpuscles and is generally harmful to the metabolic processes of the body. In fact, alcohol is a poison with the very word "intoxicated" meaning "poisoned." And yet despite this knowledge there is a generally held belief that a little alcohol taken every day will open up the coronary arteries, and that, therefore, it is advisable for heart cases to take a little nip of liquor every day. Fortunately, according to revised medical opinion, this is not considered so, and it is known to be dangerous to indulge in this practice. Perhaps alcohol will generate a temporary effect, as it works as a sedative, but it would be foolish for a heart case to think that it functioned as a coronary vasodilator. If employed regularly it will only create a false sense of physical fitness and security and that could lead to fatal consequences.

**Sub-Question:** What of coffee drinking and its effect on the heart?

**Answer:** Coffee drinking is bad for the heart. Of all the harm that coffee drinking does, its ability to prevent iron from being utilized in the body is one of the more serious disadvantages. This could lead to anemia which is a rather unpleasant complication for a heart case. We see that caffeine is capable of using up important vitamins so necessary to the health of a heart case. Caffeine in coffee can create an inositol deficiency as well as biotin deficiency —both B complex vitamins. Caffeine as a drug is sometimes used by the medical profession in certain cases of heart trouble. It dilates the coronary arteries, and furnishes a better blood supply to the heart. Many heart cases will experience a sense of comfort with coffee, but this is a short term effect only. In the long run, caffeine is known to destroy nerve cells and can affect the brain. And it becomes one of those habits, dulling the senses of a lot of the organs, including the heart, and obscuring the real problem which should be tackled. A troubled heart doesn't need coffee to get it through the day. That way is just biding time. Replace the coffee habit early—who knows the cumulative effect of caffeine on an individual at later ages?—with a program of healthy living. One last thing. A heart case should be very careful how he cuts out coffee, if he has come to depend on it. If he experiences any symptoms, then he must go on a rigorous program of developing his body. Temporarily, he might reduce the number of cups a day, or drink half cups. But gradually, through careful body conditioning, he is bound to conquer the habit without distressing his heart.

**Question:** A close relative recently suffered an attack of indigestion and upon further examination found out that it was actually a heart attack. What is the connecting factor that makes indigestion something that so readily takes place in and around heart condition?

**Answer:** It is not uncommon for an individual to suffer an attack of indigestion and to find out later that it was actually a heart attack. Mistakes are made and confusion arises not only with the laymen, but also with doctors. Sometimes symptoms that occur in attacks of indigestion may stimulate such acute abdominal conditions as perforated gastric or duodenal ulcer, gallstone colic or acute pancreatitis that unless the possibility of a heart attack is kept in mind it is easy to see how the abdomen may be opened with unfortunate consequences. On the other hand, a digestive upset or an acute gallbladder attack may sometimes be mistaken for a heart attack. When these attacks subside, those involved, laymen as well as doctors, often continue under the illusion that the patient suffered from a heart attack and recovered from it. Digestive upsets often cause pressure against the heart and this in turn interferes with its functions and impedes the circulation. They contribute to a weakening or flabbiness of the heart muscle, and often lead to a dilatation or enlargement of the heart. It is true that faulty eating and harmful living habits can cause certain heart symptoms such as palpitation, heart irregularity, weakness or pain around the heart. It is essential to remember that these symptoms do not always indicate that the heart is damaged, since they can also be caused by weakened or debilitated nerves or digestive upsets. These symptoms, even when not the result of a heart condition, must nevertheless be regarded as a warning, since if permitted to continue over an extended period of time they can ultimately lead to permanent impairment of the heart. When a patient who suffers from certain distressing symptoms in the region of the heart is reassured that he is in good condition, he must still not be complacent about it, since a failure to correct the ailment responsible for these symptoms can ultimately damage the heart or bring on some other serious ailment.

**Question:** Is the use of drugs ever really of any great help to a person whose heart is already damaged?

**Answer:** No drugs actually restore health, they merely modify or suppress the symptoms of disease. This holds true with equal force to the drugs used in heart disease.

The drugs most often used in heart disease are digitalis, the mercurial diuretic, and the nitrites. Digitalis causes an increase in the contraction of the heart, and slows down the number of heartbeats per minute. This improves the circulation and provides the heart with greater intervals of rest. Needless to say, digitalis often provides dramatic relief. However, the relief is only of a temporary nature, and no permanent correction is possible unless the muscle of the heart is strengthened and rebuilt. Investigations into the effects of digitalis on the heart when used over an extended period of time reveal that this drug is a poison whose cumulative buildup in the system can cause degeneration of the heart muscle fibers and inflammatory changes.

The mercurial diuretics are drugs that force the expulsion of large quantities of fluid through the kidneys. This relieves the heart of the added strain and protects it against the danger of collapse. Tetany, uremia, stupor, and in some cases death of the patient shortly after injection are known reactions to the use of the mercurial diuretics. Also, the administration of the mercurials leads to the excretion of many other essential elements, to the diminution of the alkalinity of the body, and to a disturbance in the balance between sodium and potassium that leads to a preponderance of potassium in the system. And potassium intoxication results in widespread impairment of neuromuscular function causing mortality and morbidity.

The nitrites (nitroglycerin and amyl nitrite) relieve severe angina attacks most dramatically. You just place a pellet of nitroglycerin under your tongue or break one of the tablets of amyl nitrite in your handkerchief and breathe it. The attack subsides immediately. This is accomplished by the nitrites forcing the heart to work harder while helping to dilate the arteries. This lowers the blood pressure and relieves the attack. Again, realize here how the basic condition is still not changed, no matter how welcome the relief may be. It is important to mention that as the use of these remedies is continued, the attacks often recur with more frequency and greater severity. Many sufferers who start with one nitroglycerin tablet occasionally will end up with a constant need, sometimes taking them as often as every 15 minutes. Physicians know that nitrites will combine with the body's oxygen and reduce its availability for function use. Thus, a vicious circle is established.

If all these drugs are ultimately inadvisable, our first objective in conjunction with getting away from their use would be to improve circulation to the heart, and to overcome the periodic spasms that cause these attacks. A program that embodies the use of simple, natural, easily digestible foods, and a restricted dietary regimen, even complete with plenty of rest, can work wonders. This is a sound approach and should be followed in all types of heart disease. In those cases where digitalis and the mercurial diuretics have been used routinely and where, because of the patient's condition, cannot be discontinued immediately or completely, this basic approach will help to strengthen and rebuild the damaged and weakened heart and reduce the need for them, and in many cases, may ultimately make their use entirely unnecessary. There are many cases where mercurial diuretics were used as often as two or three times a week but where by eliminating food for short periods of time and reducing the fluid intake, plus proper nursing care, the need for them was considerably reduced or the patient was able to do without them altogether.

**Question:** What of physical exercise—too much and/or too little—and heart disease?

**Answer:** The outdoor life and physical exercises, indulged in properly and used in conjunction with the other wholesome habits of living, will provide a well-rounded program of healthful living and serve as an added protection against the onset of heart diseases. This is now being recognized by an ever greater number of authorities. Outdoor sports and physical exercises promote the intake of oxygen into the lungs, counteract stagnation, strengthen the abdominal muscles, and increase the blood supply to the heart, and in this way do much to strengthen the heart and the blood vessels. Of course, this does not mean that one can gorge himself on rich indigestible foods or that he can wear himself out in business and social activities and think that long walks or a Sunday spent on the links will undo harm. There must be a balance and particularly as it applies to heart diseases, physical exercise must fit into all aspects of healthy living. Never indulge in exercise indiscriminately and make sure that you follow only those exercises which have been outlined for you to meet particular needs. If you are a very weak or debilitated person the best exercise would be done in a reclining position since this induces more complete relaxation and is least taxing to the heart. Never exercise to the point of fatigue, stopping before you are very tired. If tired, then stop, take deep slow breaths, and rest, before continuing to exercise. Do the exercises simply and whenever possible perform the exercises on a hard surface or on the floor. And avoid competitive sports. One need not spend hours in daily calisthenics. Walking furnishes a very interesting form of exercise, although at least 10 minutes of daily setting-up exercises can be very valuable. It was once thought that exercise or severe activity led to heart attack. Now it is believed that proper exercise is actually a form of insurance to prevent a heart attack. A man may do in safety anything he can do in comfort and he is well advised to remain active within his limits of comfortable exertion, rather than sink into himself and lead a life of invalidism. If he remains active, the development of the collateral circulation is assisted by the increased blood flow which accompanies effort. There isn't a part of the body that doesn't seem to be aided by exercise and muscular activity.

**Question:** Apart from a general exercise program, what about walking each and every day for the heart? Is that essential?

**Answer:** Movement, every day, is what the heart needs. Some people say that they are so busy that they are not certain when they will have time to walk. Well, squeeze the time in somehow. Everything else will get done. Here is an interesting plan for the beginning walker. Start off by walking 15 minutes before going to work. Then do 15 minutes during the lunch period, and 15 minutes before or after the evening meal. Slowly these periods can be lengthened until one finds that he is doing two hours a day without any trouble at all. If there is something about your kind of heart condition that you think contra-indicates walking, you will know it after your first 15 minutes. But it would be best to clear it with your doctor first—and then follow some kind of plan. At the beginning it would be best to search out a flat terrain, otherwise heart cases will experience angina symptoms. You will probably have more difficulty at the beginning of a walk than in the second half. If pressure pains occur, rest a moment or two. At the beginning of muscular exertion, time is required for the adjustment of the circulation to the increased oxygen demands. But this initial period of oxygen deficiency soon passes. The taking of vitamin E, which increases the oxygenation of the body, is very helpful to walkers. There is a great advantage to heart cases in walking regularly, rather than merely at weekends. Give the heart a daily treatment. It is just like taking vitamins—you must do it every day. The cumulative effect on the heart's action will soon be noticeable. After a while you will develop a kinesthetic sense, that is, a sense of surefootedness, a sense of perception of muscular movement. It will create grace in the motions of the body. Here are a few cautions against walking. If you walk in the sun, do not wear rimless glasses. Have glasses with dark rims. Cancer of the skin has been caused by the sun penetrating through the unrimmed glass and shining on the skin in the manner of a magnifying glass, which, by means of the sun's rays, can set fire to a piece of paper. Also if walking in the city you must be aware of the streets which are polluted with gasoline and chimney vapors. Therefore, if the country or large parks are not available, and you are forced to walk in the city, take large doses of rose hip vitamin C and desiccated liver. These are known to aid the body in getting rid of toxic substances. If you have a highly nutritious diet, if you indulge in plenty of walking and do everything possible to harden your body and make it healthy, the polluted air should do somewhat less harm to you. In walking, keep your head up, don't drag your feet on the ground and do not keep your feet too far apart. And with the sun shining up above, you've got to develop a walking program with moderation in regard to very bright days. Get a reasonable amount of sunlight, but at times choose the shady side of the road, or wear a protective covering for your head. In some cases too much sun has attacked the nose, creating tiny pimples which could by symptoms of something more serious. If you walk a lot, you will become a happier as well as a healthier person. It is a remarkable tonic for the nervous system. Unhappy people who go to psychiatrists should try walking. It is far better medicine for the sick of mind and for those with sick hearts. Walking is nearly as important as food.

**Question:** Can such a minor form of sickness as the common cold affect the heart to any great degree?

**Answer:** It has been shown that any infection in patients with heart disease is hazardous and demands prompt treatment or prevention. This includes the infection known as the common cold. Respiratory infections, particularly colds, can be irritating and aggravating factors in congestive heart failure. Any sort of respiratory infection in the person with a weak heart may initiate cardiac failure by causing damage to the heart muscle or by favoring congestion of the lungs. Therefore it is most important to look for and treat respiratory infection in cardiac patients. To prevent colds, practically no bread or other rye or wheat products should be eaten. The elimination of wheat and rye products goes a long way towards the complete annihilation of the common cold. Another preventive measure for the congestive heart failure patient is the taking of vitamins A and D in the form of halibut liver oil. This has the effect of strengthening the mucous membranes all over the body. When this happens in the nasal regions, it makes it that much more difficult for disease germs to breed there. But of all the vitamins, C is the most important in the prevention of colds. And vitamin C cannot only prevent colds, but if given in tremendous amounts after a cold has started, can abort it within an hour or two. If we are talking about the heart and disease and we are aware that the common cold is known to have a direct relation to the frequent occurrence of heart failure among cardiac patients, the particular heart victim should at least obey the simple diet and vitamin rules to insure that the possibilities of respiratory infection are reduced to a minimum. The amazing part of all this is the fact that so many of the things that will prevent colds are also good to keep the action of the heart healthy.

## BIBLIOGRAPHY

Bailey, Herbert, *Vitamin E: Your Key to a Healthy Heart*, Arc Books, Inc.

Fraser, Harris D., *The Man Who Discovered the Circulation of Blood*, Popular Science Monthly Pub.

Nuzum, Franklin Richards, *The Span of Life as Influenced By the Heart, the Kidneys and the Blood Vessels*, C. C. Thomas & Co.

Poynter, C. W.M., *Congenital Anomalies of the Arteries and Veins of the Human Body*, University of Nebraska Press.

Rodale, J. I. and Staff, *Encyclopedia of Common Diseases*, Rodale Books, Inc.

Shepard, John Frederick, *The Circulation and Sleep*, Macmillan Co.

Snyder, Eugene F., *From a Doctor's Heart*, Philosophical Library.

Stuart, Jesse, *The Year of My Rebirth*, McGraw-Hill.

Sydenstricker, Edgar, *Health and Environment*, McGraw-Hill.

Waldo, Myra, *Cooking for Your Heart and Health*, Putnam.

Warmbrand, Max, *Add Years to Your Heart*, Pyramid Books.

# CANCER

**Question:** When one hears that cancer is growing in the body what, in technical terms, does that exactly mean?

**Answer:** To explore the complex world of cancer it would be wise to know what is physically happening in the cells and tissues of a body in which cancer is taking place. Cancer is an abnormal and unrestrained new growth in cells and tissues that produces injurious and often fatal results. Cells and tissues are said to be cancerous when, for no known reason, they grow more rapidly than normal, assume abnormal shapes and sizes and cease functioning in a normal manner. The ultimate involvement of a vital organ by cancer, either primary or metastatic (transitory), may lead to the death of the patient. Cancer in contrast to tumors tends to spread into contiguous tissues and also metastasize. In metastasis, cancerous cells break off from the original lesion and are carried in the blood where they set up new lesions. Cancer is said to be malignant because of its tendency to cause death if not treated. Benign tumors usually do not cause death, although they may, if they interfere with a normal body function by virtue of the location or size.

In general, cancer cells divide at a higher rate than do normal cells, but this is not always true; for example, in the organization of the callus in a fractured bone and in the relining of the uterus by endometrium after menstruation, the normal cells divide at a higher rate than do the cancer cells. It is true also, that some malignant tumors have intermittent growth and latent periods. The distinction between the growth of cancerous and normal tissues is not so much the rapidity of cell division in the former as it is the partial or complete loss of growth restraint in cancer cells and their failure to metamorphose into a useful, limited tissue of the type that characterizes the functional equilibrium of growth of normal tissue. Cancer may not be so autonomous as once was believed. The lesions probably are influenced by the host's susceptibility and immunity. Certain cancers of the breast and prostate, for example, are considered dependent on hormones for their

137

existence; other cancers are dependent on the presence of specific viruses.

It should be pointed out now that cancer is not merely a medical problem: it is a biological phenomenon, whose elucidation is bound up with advances in a number of key fields of present day biology. Like most biological phenomena it is multi-causal: there is no single cause of cancer. The disease is not a biological entity, like chromosomes or paratyphoid B, or natural groups such as Insecta or Amphibia. It merely denotes a category; the term cancer is a convenient label or pigeon-hole for a number of pathological tissue-conditions exhibiting certain common characteristics, but all unique in certain other respects. Indeed it is not "a" disease at all but an assemblage of many different diseases which have certain symptoms in common. A century ago, medical men spoke of "fever" as a disease. Now they no longer do so. Something of the sort is happening with cancer during the present century.

**Question:** How is the cancer that is growing in the body identified?

**Answer:** At least 50 percent of all cancers are visible on inspection, or can be reached for palpation by an examining finger; at least 25 percent more can be seen with special examining instruments that are inserted within the orifices of the body.

The first of three steps in diagnosis is a careful elicitation of the patient's complaints relating to abnormalities in the functioning of a specific organ. The symptom complex elaborated by most cancers is sufficiently characteristic to arouse the physician's suspicion when recited by the patient. The second step is a careful physical examination that leads in most cases to the discovery of the malignant tumor and a recognition of its extent and character. By using special hollow instruments that are electrically illuminated and equipped with magnifying lenses, the examining physician is able to inspect the lower colon, rectum, urinary bladder, larynx, bronchi and gullet. This procedure is referred to generally as endoscopy and specifically as they relate to the organs just listed as laryngoscopy, bronchoscopy, esophagoscopy, gastroscopy, proctoscopy and cystoscopy. X-ray study, with or without the utilization of contrasting media, is important in the diagnosis of cancers within the nasal sinuses, lungs, esophagus, stomach, colon, intestines, kidneys, bladder, bone and brain. Chemical tests for cancer were generally discarded soon after being proposed, but a few for special types of cancer are valid, such as those for an increased acid phosphatase content of the blood in patients with cancer of the prostate and a quantitative increase of albumoses in the blood and urine of patients with myeloma. The final step in establishing the diagnosis is the biopsy, in which a portion of the suspected cancerous tissue is removed for microscopic study and identification. The microscopic characteristics of various cancers are so definite and well known that this method serves as an accurate check on the diagnosis and usually enables the examiner to identify the tissue or organ of origin. Specimens for biopsy are removed by forceps or electric snare, or a plug of tissue is obtained by syringe aspiration, or cells may be obtained from body fluids, such as uterine, vaginal, gastric, bronchial or urinary secretions.

**Question:** Is there any simple method of classification of the different kinds of cancer?

**Answer:** There are two types of cancer according to the simplest methods of classification—that of calling the cancer a carcinoma or sarcoma depending on whether the cancer originated in epithelial or nonepithelial tissue. The latter term refers chiefly to the structural framework of the body, including muscle, fat, connective tissue, bone cartilage, tendon, etc. It follows, therefore, that as many varieties of cancer exist as there are organs and tissues within the body. Each type and subtype of cancer has its own histological appearance and can be identified by microscopic study; the behavior or natural history of each type has been well determined so that the pathologist can predict the manner of its growth.

Cancers may also be classified according to the stage of the disease; for example: (1) early, or localized, when still confined to the tissue of origin (frequently curable); (2) metastatic, or spread to regional lymph nodes, or invading contagious structures (sometimes curable); and (3) widely disseminated throughout the body (usually incurable).

Cancers can also be classified into one of four grades on the basis of their degree of malignancy, as determined by microscopic examination. Grade one cancers (barely malignant) tend to differentiate toward and resemble the cells of the tissue of origin, whereas grade four cancers (highly malignant) are composed of cells extremely active in cell division. The other two grades represent intermediate degrees of differentiation and reproduction. It follows that grade four cancers as a rule grow more rapidly, metastasize earlier and more widely, pursue a more rapid course and have lower rate of curability than the other three grades.

**Question:** Are there certain diseases that are considered particularly dangerous because they can lead to or are followed by cancer?

**Answer:** Yes there are certain diseases and conditions that are considered precancerous. Malignant tumors do not develop inevitably but occur with such frequency that the term precancerous has been applied to these conditions. An example is the presence of gallstones; the incidence in gallbladders is approximately 5 percent of the general population. But 98 percent of the persons who develop cancer of the gallbladder have or have had gallstones, which is a strong indication that the chronic irritation of the stones is a causative factor of the cancer. Leukoplakia, another example, is a disease in which thick, white patches appear on the mucous membrane of the tongue, lips, cheek, floor of the mouth palate, tonsil or other mucosa-lined organs such as the male and female genitals and the esophagus. Cancer of the type known as epidermoid or squamous cell carcinoma develops with some frequency in those locations, probably because of pre-existing leukoplakia. Syphilis of the tongue sometimes predisposes to the development of lingual cancer; in fact 25 percent of all patients who have cancer within the oral cavity have had syphilis, which is a higher incidence by far than in the general population. The neck of the womb may subsequently become cancerous if badly scarred, eroded or chronically infected, as sometimes occurs sequential to childbirth. Certain benign tumors are precancerous in varying percentages; examples are benign adenomas of the thyroid gland, polyps of the colon, papillomas of the urinary bladder and the common pigmented mole of the skin. Radiation dermatitis caused by overexposure of the skin to x-rays, as when improper dosages are used to treat acne or excess hair on the face, also may be precancerous. Keratoses, which are warty overgrowths of the skin occurring in elderly persons or persons with oily skin, may degenerate over joints so that scar cancers develop. The scarred skin lacks the oil glands and the elastic tissue that normally protect the skin against irritation. The early grafting of new skin in burns lessens the incidence of scar cancers later. Certain types of mastitis, when accompanied by overgrowth of the ductal elements, may under certain conditions become cancerous.

**Question:** Can you give me the symptoms and course of certain of the more common cancers?

**Answer:** This widely asked question will be answered by breaking down the various parts of the body and discussing the cancers as they are related to the individual parts. This will give you a more thorough and specific view, all in one. And will hopefully provide documentation on a simple and easily understandable level.

**Sub-Question:** What of cancer of the skin?

**Answer:** Cancer of the skin may appear as a progressively enlarging ulcer with hard, elevated margins and no tendency to heal spontaneously. Pain is conspicuously absent in many cases until the disease becomes advanced. It appears in other forms as a horny overgrowth of skin or as a fissure that generates in a scar. Between 75 and 95 percent of all the cases can be cured. Half of the cases of malignant melanoma develop from pre-existing pigmented moles and the other half from apparently intact skin. It is the most malignant of all accessible cancers and soon metastasizes through both lymphatic and blood vessels to lymph nodes and internal organs. The cure rate is seldom higher than 70 percent of cases treated, depending on the presence or absence of metastases.

**Sub-Question:** What of cancer of the oral cavity?

**Answer:** Cancers of the lower lip develop as fissures, elevated plaques of keratosis or hard ulcers situated on the vermilion border, usually of the lower lip. At least 90 percent of these cancers are cured if treated before metastases develop. Cancer of the tongue appears as a fissure, chronic ulcer or indurated segment of the tongue, commonly on the lateral or posterior margins. It is one of the few cancers that is painful in its early stages and consequently is recognized early because of its tenderness and interference with the mobility of the tongue. Extension of the cancer to the lymph nodes in the neck occurs relatively early because of the high grade of malignancy of this type of cancer and the rich lymph drainage of the tongue. The cure rate is seldom above 22 to 30 percent of patients treated. Cancer of the larynx may be detected early by an investigation of persistent hoarseness or changes in the voice. The development of difficult breathing is an indication of an advanced stage of the disease. The prognosis of cancer of the larynx is good following radiological treatment or surgical removal of the larynx.

**Sub-Question:** What of cancer of the thyroid gland?

**Answer:** Cancer of the thyroid gland requires surgical removal of the gland and of the lymph nodes on the same side of the neck as the cancerous lesion. All nodular goiters, as distinguished from smooth enlargements and those associated with the toxic symptoms of hyperthyroidism, require immediate surgical removal because these nodules, even though painless, inconspicuous and without symptoms, are found on subsequent microscopic study to be cancerous in 8 to 20 percent of cases.

**Sub-Question:** What of cancer of the neck?

**Answer:** Cancer of the neck is usually secondary to a primary cancer in the mouth, pharynx, larynx, hypopharynx, chest or abdomen; less frequently, the primary site is within the structures of the neck. The appearance of a lump in the neck, if the thyroid gland is excluded from consideration, should arouse suspicion of a possible undetected and symptomatic cancer within the mouth or adjacent structures, and it calls for careful investigation to discover the site of origin. When found, it requires treatment of the primary cancer and of the metastatic cancer within the cervical lymph nodes by radical surgical excision with or without irradiation by X-rays and radium.

**Sub-Question:** What of cancer of the lung?

**Answer:** Cancer of the lung was apparently increasing in frequency in the mid-1960's, partly because of improvements in diagnosis and partly because of an increment in occurrence of the disease. Its presence is heralded by the onset of a cough that persists and may not be productive until later when expectoration of blood occurs. Its true character can be identified by X-ray study supplemented by bronchoscopic visualization and biopsy. The removal of the entire lung with dissection of those lymph nodes in the mediastinum that drain the lung offers opportunities for cure that formerly did not exist.

**Sub-Question:** What of cancer of the esophagus?

**Answer:** Cancer of the esophagus causes progressively increasing difficulty in swallowing, chiefly of course with solid foods. The patient voluntarily ingests a diet that is soft and liquid; diagnosis can be established by X-ray study, esophagoscopy and biopsy. The esophagus may be removed partially or completely; it can be replaced partially or completely by a joining together (anastomosis) in the chest of the remaining sections or by elevating the stomach and joining a remaining section to it or by interposing a section of colon between the remnants of the esophagus at the base of the neck.

**Sub-Question:** What of cancer of the stomach?

**Answer:** Cancers of the stomach develop insidiously and are difficult to diagnose because of the absence of specific symptoms. Gradual onset of indigestion in a person of previously good health with symptoms occasionally suggesting peptic ulcer, associated with an unexplained loss of weight, anemia, loss of appetite, and, in the advanced stages, vomiting and the presence of a mass that can be felt in the abdomen, are common diagnostic features of the disease. The diagnosis is confirmed by X-ray study and gastroscopic visualization. Because of improved, more radical surgical technique, 60 percent of cancers of the stomach became resectable and of this group 35 percent of the patients were cured.

**Sub-Question:** What of cancer of the pancreas?

**Answer:** Cancers of the pancreas are seldom diagnosed early because of the absence of localized signs and symptoms. A radical operation was designed for successful treatment, but the end results were bad because of the delayed diagnosis. The presence of unexplained deep abdominal pain with backache, occasional diarrhea and later development of jaundice with the absence of gallstones are suspicious symptoms that indicate the possible presence of this disease.

**Question:** What of cancer of the rectum?

**Answer:** Cancers of the rectum often are erroneously diagnosed as hemorrhoids in the early stages because of the frequent first symptom of repeated small hemorrhages with bowel movements. The usual indications of a rectal tumor are an incomplete sense of relief after defecation associated with some tenesmus or spasm, increased frequency of bowel movements, the passage of a mucous discharge with or without the stools and a change in the shape of the feces. Approximately 80 percent of the rectal cancers are resectable by radical operation, and about 50 percent of the operations produce permanent cures.

**Question:** What of cancer of the breast?

**Answer:** Cancer of the breast appears initially as a small, painless lump that grows in size; it subsequently may adhere to the skin, causing dimpling and later ulceration; the nipple sometimes becomes inverted. All lumps in the breast should be suspected of being cancerous until proved noncancerous. Although the disease develops more frequently in women of middle age than in any other age group, 17 percent of the cases occur in women under 40 years. One percent of all breast cancer occurs in men, chiefly those of middle and old age. Cancer of the breast metastasizes or spreads most frequently to the lymph nodes in the armpit on the corresponding side of the body and sometimes to a chain of lymph nodes beneath the junction of the sternum and the ribs; until it spreads beyond these nodes it is still operable and curable. In 78 percent of patients with cancer confined to the breast, a cure is obtained by removing the breast, muscles of the chest wall and the regional lymph nodes; 42 percent of patients who have cancer of the breast with metastases to the regional lymph nodes and without evidence of dissemination elsewhere are cured by the radical operation. Cancer of the breast may spread by lymph and blood vessels to other organs, such as the lungs, the brain or the bony skeleton, under which circumstances X-ray treatment and hormone therapy are excellent palliative measures.

**Sub-Question:** What of uterine cancer?

**Answer:** Cancer of the neck (cervix) of the uterus develops most frequently in women 30 to 50 years of age but may occur before 30 or after 50. Women who develop cancer of the uterine cervix often have sustained injury to the cervix during childbirth. The onset of the disease is heralded by excessive uterine bleeding either at the time of menstruation or in the intermenstrual phase or on sexual intercourse. The discharge may be brown and foul as well as bloody; actual hemorrhages may occur. Cancer of the interior of the body of the uterus (endometrial cancer) is relatively more frequent in women who have not borne children; it occurs in a slightly older age group, usually post-menopausal. It is more difficult to diagnose than the cervical type since it is not visible. A diagnostic curettage of the uterus (obtaining a biopsy specimen with a scraping tool) may be done or secretions from the uterus may be studied for identification of cancer cells. By the proper application of X-ray and radium therapy or radical surgical excision, the curability of cancers of the uterus varies from 30 to 75 percent.

**Sub-Question:** What of cancers of the urinary bladder and kidney?

**Answer:** Cancers of the urinary bladder and kidney produce an initial symptom of blood in the urine (hematuria) that may be accompanied by frequent urination and pain. The exact location of the cancer may be determined by combined X-ray study and cystoscopic visualization of the urinary bladder. Cancers of the kidney may grow as silent tumors and may not be suspected until metastatic focuses appear in distant parts, such as the bones, lungs or brain.

**Sub-Question:** What of cancer of the prostate?

**Answer:** Cancer of the prostate in elderly men may provoke no symptoms other than occasional difficulty in micturition. Sometimes the first indication of the presence of this cancer is backache, which is caused by metastases of the prostatic cancer throughout the bones of the pelvis and vertebral column. Surgical treatment is employed only for the relief of obstruction to the urinary outflow and in rare cases for the extirpation of early cancers.

The majority of prostatic cancers are in an advanced stage when diagnosed and are treated palliatively by a combination of castration and the administration of female sex hormones or their synthetic chemical equivalents.

**Sub-Question:** What of cancer of the bone?

**Answer:** Cancer of the bone may occur in any age group, including children and young adolescents. The presence of pain and disability in an extremity, when associated with an enlargement of a bone, is a significant sign of an early bone sarcoma. Amputation, if performed early, may permit a curability in 10 to 15 percent of these patients.

**Question:** Please tell me about leukemia and its relationship to infants and young children.

**Answer:** Leukemia is cancer of the blood. There is an increase in the white blood corpuscles, and enlargement of the spleen, the lymphatic glands and the bone marrow. The incidence of leukemia has been rising all over the world in our present century. We know that it is more prevalent in males than in females and that the aged are affected and children as well. In the last 10 years, there has been an alarming increase in the incidence of leukemia in infants and young children, the cause of which has led to much investigative research and conjecture. In the United States, more children five to 14 years of age are victims of this disease than of any other, and it is invariably fatal. The view towards leukemia present at birth (congenital leukemia) holds that it is as obscure as it is in the childhood form, but that existence of this disease in the unborn child does suggest that maternal and hereditary factors significantly pertain to the cause of disease in both forms. Most newborns with signs of leukemia at birth have severe systemic involvement and die within a few years. Hemorrhagic manifestations occur in the infant ranging from small rounded spots of bleeding under the skin to bleeding from the umbilical stump, the digestive and elimination tracts.

The most generally accepted circumstance of blame for leukemia in the newborn child has been the exposure of the pregnant mother to diagnostic or therapeutic X-ray, thus exposing the unborn child to unintentional radiation. But this exposure can only be a small part of the increasing incidence in infantile subjects. Another factor is the tobacco smoking of mothers during pregnancy. Just think of the many millions of unborn progeny who are receiving the toxic elements of tobacco smoke through the mother's inhalation which leads into the bloodstream. Acute leukemia occurs chiefly before the age of 20, and it is one of the commonest forms of malignant disease in young children. It follows an active course, beginning in a stormy fashion. The lowered resistance of children with leukemia makes them ready victims of infection. And the leukemic state is often ushered in by an attack of an acute infectious illness, such as tonsilitis, a severe "cold," a boil, or an abscessed tooth. Instead of subsiding rapidly as one would expect in a simple illness, the fever continues, and the patient remains prostrated, listless and weak. For children, in the last few years, there has come a succession of new chemical compounds which singly or in combination cause remissions of disease. They are not successful in every case, nor can their success be predicted. But they help often enough to be hailed by patients, parents and doctors. At present there are only a few of these new drugs. And the use of some of them is still restricted because of their experimental nature. Properly selected and administered they will interrupt the headlong course of disease in about two-thirds of the youngsters. Thanks to them, over half of all little leukemia patients are now permitted to live a year or more after the illness begins—some of them for several years. Small gain, perhaps. But certainly a precious one to all parents of these children. And a gain that brightens the hopes of everyone—doctors and scientists most of all—that permanently effective drugs are in the offing.

There is at present no cure for leukemia in reference to any sex, any age. But watchful care of patients and treatment at appropriate intervals will relieve its distressing symptoms and signs for varying lengths of time and will thereby maintain the patient in an active condition for the longest possible time. Treatment for leukemia consists of X-rays applied to major areas of disease activity—the spleen, enlarged lymph nodes, and selected bones. Within the past 15 years, radioactive isotopes—usually radiophosphorus—have been administered by mouth or injection into the bloodstream. The results have been good in certain types of the disease. More recently, a few chemicals have come into general use—notably ACTH and cortisone, which increase the effectiveness of irradiation therapy in the later stages of disease or in more resistant cases. Often these new drugs restore the patient to apparent health for a while even after X-rays appear to have lost their effectiveness. But they must be used with extreme caution.

**Question:** Please tell me about viruses and their possibilities as cancer-causing agents.

**Answer:** We can talk about viruses and cancers basically in terms of what has been learned about the subject through experimentation with animals. We know that several kinds of tumor, benign and malignant, that occur in animals are due to viruses— those strange agents of disease so small that they pass through porcelain and are visible only under the extremely powerful electron miscroscope. Viruses are the cause of a warty tumor of the skin, affecting wild rabbits, and of another tumor of the skin, this one malignant, that also occurs in rabbits. A cancer of the kidney sometimes found in frogs is caused by a virus, and so is a leukemia-like disease of the blood affecting chickens and other fowl. The first tumor ever shown to be caused by a virus was the chicken sarcoma, which was discovered in 1910 to be transmissible from an infected bird to a healthy one under the circumstances that made a virus the most likely suspect—even though no one had ever actually seen a virus. Within the past few years, evidence has suggested that leukemia in certain strains of mice may be induced by viruses, as may be a tumor involving the salivary glands of the same species.

Recently, many reesarchers have turned their attention to the role of a particular agent that behaves like a virus. This agent seems to have an important influence—probably the determining one—in the appearance of cancer in the breast of mice. It is transmitted from mother to offspring in the mother's milk, and some investigators say that it has the physical structure of a virus as seen in the electron microscope. In this way, the "milk factor," as the infecting agent is called, is passed along through succeeding generations of mice. When it is present in a strain or "breed" of mice, cancer of the breast will develop in about eight or nine out of every

10 females that live long enough to get it. But if the newborn female offspring are removed from their mother immediately after birth—before they have nursed at her breasts even once—and are placed with a foster mother of a strain that does not carry the "milk factor," they will not develop cancer as they grow older—or will do so only rarely. There is no direct evidence that the "milk factor" causes cancer of the breast in human beings, but a few scientists believe that such a possibility may exist. Although they have not accepted the existence of a transmissible agent as the cause of human cancer of the breast, the discovery of the "milk factor" and of other viruslike substances responsible for certain tumors in animals has revived the interest of scientists in viruses and in their possible relation to tumor growth in general and cancer in humans specifically.

**Question:** In recently moving to a warm climate I find myself relaxing on the beach constantly, enjoying the rays of the sun. Is this exposure in any way a possible cause of cancer?

**Answer:** Repeated sunburn, although many people do not want to admit it, is perhaps the most widespread of the known causes of cancer. Long exposure to strong sunlight seems to be much more likely to cause skin cancer in people of certain complexions than in others, and the rate of cancer of the skin varies directly with the amount of sunlight received in any given place. It occurs most often among those who are constantly exposed to the sun, and usually in the unprotected parts of the body—the face, neck, forearms and the hands. The connection between sunlight and skin cancer is so striking the disease long ago was dubbed "sailor's cancer" or "farmer's cancer."

On the subject of rays, don't overlook the harmfulness of being an inside "sun" worshipper. Namely, it has been proven that ultraviolet rays generated by the misuse of sunlamps can serve to cause cancer. In speaking about the sun we are talking about radiation and here would be a good place to discuss other kinds of radiation that may cause cancer, too. X-rays and the rays of radium can restrain and destroy cancer, but they can also cause it. It all depends on how big a dose a person gets. In the early days of the use of these rays in diagnosis and treatment, before we knew what the safe limits of exposure were, many physicians overexposed themselves, especially their hands. Later they developed cancer of the skin. The hazard still exists for physicians who specialize in X-ray diagnostic work, and who use the fluoroscope extensively. Inevitably, these specialists receive some of the penetrating beams of X-rays over large areas of the body. Recently we have heard a great deal about the experimental, commercial and medical uses of radioactive isotopes. There are similar dangers here, although the problem was recognized beforehand and from the start all possible safeguards were set up to protect personnel handling such materials and patients being treated with them.

The medical branches of the Armed Forces have been intensely interested in the survivors of the atomic explosions at Hiroshima and Nagasaki, for it seemed probable that some of these Japanese had been exposed to amounts of high-intensity radiation sufficient to result in leukemia and perhaps other cancer-related conditions as time went on. And now we know that they were!

Cosmic rays are extremely short-wave, very penetrating, radiations which bombard the earth constantly from outer space. The effects of cosmic rays on living things are not yet understood. But, since they are relatives of X-rays, the suggestion has been made that they may be partly responsible for cancer among humans and animals. However, there is no way of avoiding them—except to live many feet beneath the earth's surface. So there is not much to be gained by worrying about them. Actually, certain statistics seem to deny that cosmic rays are an important cause of cancer. For example, cancer occurs at least as often in the low coastal regions of the East as it does in high Rocky Mountain plateaus— where cosmic rays are much more numerous.

**Question:** Can you tell me more about diet—what people eat or do not eat—and what bearing this all has on causing cancers to grow?

**Answer:** The question of diet has proved quite controversial. Of course, we know that nutrition is important to a healthy body, but some physicians feel that cancer does not appear as a result of dietary factors and in general cannot be prevented or cured by dietary rules. Still, it is agreed that there are several items in the human diet which do seem related to certain kinds of cancer. Also a look at oxidation-enzymes and vitamins does reveal interesting theories to back up the feelings of those who believe nutrition to play a more vital role in generating cancers.

Arsenic, for one, is related to certain kinds of cancer. It is generally found in the soil and in water, only in traces. Now, arsenic is most likely to be deposited in the skin. And some authorities say that this is the reason for the frequent skin cancers to be seen in areas of the world—like Germany and Argentina—where the arsenic content of the natural water is known to be high. The curious affinity of arsenic for the skin led to its use in medicines for treating certain skin disorders. Over a long period, enough arsenic accumulated in some patients thus treated to cause skin cancer.

A few items of the normal human diet are causes of cancer "in reverse"—that is, cancer results from their absence. One of these substances is iodine, which is essential to the normal functioning of the thyroid gland, located in the forepart of the lower neck. In most parts of the world the amount of iodine in the soil (and food grown in the soil) and in the drinking water is enough for the thyroids' requirements. But there are a few places where iodine is absent, or nearly so, from the soil and water, and here the amount taken in by humans is inadequate. Under these conditions the thyroid becomes considerably enlarged, a condition known as goiter. Goiter is benign, but most doctors feel that cancer is more likely to develop in a goiter than in a normal thyroid gland. It has been claimed that cancer of the thyroid is four times commoner in goiter regions (Switzerland, for instance) than it is elsewhere. Today, people are learning that they can prevent goiter in iodine-low regions by using iodized salt at the table and in cooking.

The much-advertised vitamin B is another item of diet that is related to cancer. Actually, vitamin B is a combination of a dozen or so food elements. It plays an important part in maintaining the health of the mucous membranes of the mouth, throat, esophagus and perhaps other areas. When there is a serious deficiency of vitamine B in the diet, the lips are likely to become dry, scaly, cracked or superficially ulcerated, and leukoplakia frequently appears. Inside the mouth, in the throat, and in the esophagus, similar changes occur. Fresh fruits and vegetables are the major sources of the vitamin. And these rare delicacies in some parts of the world—notably northernmost parts of the Scandinavian countries—indicate a relationship between the normal intake of B and cancer.

Cancer of the esophagus and of the pharynx occurs more frequently among the residents of northern Sweden and Norway than it does elsewhere in the world. This fact specifically can be attributed to the lack of the vitamin B complex.

The separation from nature has put man all over the world into overcrowded city-dwellings, in association with civilization-dictated ways of living, and he must adopt a diet accordingly. The cooking often results in a deficiency of chlorophyll and consequently a deficiency in all the products which chlorophyll assists in manufacturing in the body. All living things require oxygen which, by the process of oxidation, changes food into energy and growth. This process is aided by the presence of chlorophyll. If little or no chlorophyll is present, all the other substances created or influenced by it in this very complex process are also deficient. These substances are called oxidation-enzymes. The result, therefore, is an impoverishment of the organism in the vital-oxidation-enzymes and in the vitamins, especially C. Cancer cells always show a complete absence of vitamin C.

A condition of deficient oxygen often exists not only in cancer cells but in pre-cancerous ones and in the total organism as well. As a result of this, the molecules of protein in the cells regroup themselves and become instead giant virus molecules. So even without an actual virus infection, a formation of a virus is possible simply because of a deficiency of the various oxidation-enzymes. In addition to the oxidation-enzymes, the vitamins have a great significance in the origin of cancer. Cancer cells lack vitamin C, B and A. Cancerous and even pre-cancerous organisms have a terrific deficiency in them. Through a continued deficiency of vitamin A, an idleness in vitamin C supply occurs and the vitamin C is not replaced quickly enough. Hence a deficiency in vitamin C will always exist. The presence of vitamin C is of utmost importance in the entire oxidation process that takes place in the cells. Vitamin A is also important, for the presence of vitamin A brings about the decomposition of certain fatty acids. Through a deficiency in vitamin A the increase of these fatty acids in cancer cells can be explained.

**Sub-Question:** What about chemical substances added to food. Can they cause cancer?

**Answer:** Chemical substances that are added to food, candy, soft drinks, and other products for the purpose of coloring, flavoring, sweetening, preserving and moistening have been talked about as possible cancer-inciters. Included in a discussion of chemical additives should be the mention of insecticides, which are usually grouped under food additives even though they are not added intentionally and are not supposed to reach the consumer in harmful amounts.

Dulcin, a sweetening agent, will serve as a good example here. For many years dulcin was readily obtainable and widely used. Several years ago, however, studies of the long-term effects of dulcin showed that it caused tumors of the liver in rats. It was then promptly withdrawn from sale. It should be noted that other artificial sweeteners now on the market, such as saccharin, are harmless. Benign tumors of the liver appear to have been produced in experimental animals after prolonged feeding on chlorophenothane (DDT). Particularly interesting are certain aniline dyes that are used as coloring agents in food, soft drinks and preserves that have been shown to cause tumors under special experimental conditions. Thus, paradimethylaminoazobenzene—called "butter yellow" for short (thank goodness)—was once used in the United States to improve the eye appeal of certain foods—though not butter, strange to say. But there is now clear proof that prolonged feeding of butter yellow to mice, rats and dogs that are, at the same time, kept on a deficient vitamin B intake, will result in tumors of the liver—and less frequently of other organs. It should be noted here, as well, that currently used butter colorants, such as carotene, are certified as safe. Several other food dyes related to butter yellow are now known to cause similar effects when administered experimentally. Other food dyes belonging to a different chemical family (light green SF, brilliant blue FCF, fast green FCF) will produce malignant tumors at the site of injection into the skin of the rat beneath the surface. One important point: the dyes referred to here are manmade—that is, synthetic. There is no reason whatever to suspect pigments derived from plants—that is, the vegetable dyes.

**Question:** I've certainly heard enough connecting smoking (the "cigarettes may be hazardous to your health" line) and lung cancer. But what exactly are the effects of tobacco on the lung? I would like more detail here.

**Answer:** Numerous observations, some of them made 60 and 70 years ago, have persuaded many doctors that cancers of the lip and mouth are more likely to develop in smokers of pipes and cigars than in non-smokers. Just how smoking actually causes cancer of the tongue, the floor of the mouth, the palate, or the cheek has never been demonstrated to everyone's satisfaction. A good many hold that smoke has never been "proved" to be a cause of cancer. And yet it is indeed true that smoke, as such, has not yet been made to produce cancer. But we do know that there are at least three possible explanations of the cancer-causing effect of smoke in the mouth. First, the heat of the smoke is greatest in the mouth, and most of the heat is dissipated there. And we know that localized, repeated application of heat does cause irritation, which in turn favors the development of cancer. Second, the smoke may contain one or more cancer-causing substances, such as the complex molecules known as hydro-carbons (some of which do cause cancer). And third, even if no known cancer-causing chemical compounds had been identified in tobacco smoke, smoke might still cause cancer through the mild irritation it causes when in contact with living tissues—especially delicate ones.

Recent investigations of chewing tobacco as a possible factor in cancer of the mouth and stomach have shown that cancer of the mouth is more common in chewers than in non-chewers. But the habit seems to have little relation to cancer of the stomach, possibly because the juice is considerably diluted by the stomach secretions.

The case against smoking is directed principally at cigarettes, since almost all of the phenomenal increase in tobacco consumption in the past forty years is accounted for by cigarettes. The per capita consumption of cigars and pipe tobacco has actually dropped in the last forty years. Another telling argument is that cigarette smoke is generally inhaled into the lungs, whereas cigar and pipe smoke usually are not. The evidence is that the association of lung cancer with cigarette smoking is much stronger than it is with cigar and pipe smoking. The risk of developing lung cancer appears to increase with the amount smoked. "Amount smoked" would of course be related to the quantity smoked per day as well as to the duration of the practice—that is, the number of years involved. For example, cancer of the lung appeared more frequently in those who had begun to smoke prior to age 15 than in those who took it up after 25. Where information about inhaling was sought, the results tended to give it weight as a factor in inducing cancer: persistent deep inhalers appeared more prone to lung cancer. It has been shown that the lungs of those who smoked cigarettes indicate tissue and cell abnormalities much oftener than the lungs of those who have not. These changes consist of alterations in the structure of surface cells lining the bronchial tubes; thickening of the cell layers of the tubes and nests of deformed (cancerlike) cells. There is, moreover, reason to believe that many of the abnormalities noted in the lung tissues of cigarette smokers are precancerous. Tobacco smoke consists of an astonishing number of substances, of an astonishing number of kinds, including proteins, starches, alkaloids, hydro-carbons, phenols, fatty acids, sterols and inorganic minerals. Of particular interest has been the identification of seven compounds (called polycyclic hydrocarbons because their molecules consist of many "rings" of hydrogen and carbon atoms) which are carcinogens—that is, they can produce cancer under certain circumstances. Mouse skin-painting experiments have shown that the cancer-inducing power of cigarette tar is a good deal greater than that of any of its cancer-inducing components. One explanation of this paradox is that the tar contains substances which are not themselves producers of cancer, but which enhance the cancer causing effects of other carcinogenic compounds. They have been termed co-carcinogens.

In summary, the possible relationships between smoking and such other forms of cancer as cancer of the mouth, larynx, esophagus, and bladder; and between smoking and such non-cancerous diseases as chronic bronchitis, emphysema, stomach ulcers, and coronary artery disease are to be considered. In some instances the relationship is such that it is a question whether smoking is causally related. But there is no question whatever about the overriding evidence that the relationship between lung cancer and cigarette smoking is substantial and is causal.

**Question:** Is it true that there can be a susceptibility to cancer based on one's occupation?

**Answer:** There is a special class of environmental influences that involve only those who work in certain occupations. These are called occupational influences, and the cancers resulting from them are called occupational cancers. Although these occupational influences affect only certain groups rather than the public at large, they are of particular interest for several reasons. In the first place, they include the oldest well-established causes of cancer. Secondly, they include some of the most firmly proved causes of cancer. Finally, more and more industrial workers are being exposed to an increasing variety of new and complex chemical substances, the long-range effects of which must be carefully watched. Perhaps the first valid observation of the association between an occupation and cancer was made in 1775, when it was suggested that coal soot might in some way be responsible for cancer of the scrotum. This disease was found very frequently among chimney sweeps. The soft coal commonly burned in England gave off large quantities of soot, which had to be brushed out of the flues in order to keep them open. The "sweeps" who did the work became covered with coal soot and, since body baths were rare in those days, the soot remained in prolonged contact with the skin and accumulated especially in the folds of the scrotum. The resulting disease had long been known as "chimney sweep's cancer." So coal soot became the father of a long line of chemical substances to be identified or produced later—each of which would cause cancer of one kind or another. Years later, and not until the discovery of radioactivity and its effects on living tissues could scientists point to the precise association between working in coal mines and lung trouble. The ores in these mines are rich in pitchblende—containing relatively large amounts of strongly radioactive radium and uranium. In fact, now we know that the air in these mines contains a fine radioactive dust. Inhaled over a period of years, this dust will produce cancer of the lungs—just as excessive exposure to radium and X-rays among physicians of a generation ago resulted in cancer of the skin. In general, the occupation agents known to cause cancer do so only in specific organs of the body. The list of well-established or proved causes of occupational hazard is impressive. Arsenic, tar, creosote oil, crude paraffin oil, ionizing radiation (X-rays, radium) and sunlight can, if the contact is intense enough and long enough, result in skin cancer. Asbestos, chromate compounds, nickel carbonyl, tar fumes, and ionizing radiation increase the likelihood of cancer of the lung. Nickel carbonyl, isopropyl oil (not to be confused with isopropyl alcohol, which is made from it) and radioactive dusts and gases are accepted causes of cancer of the nasopharynx and sinuses. Aromatic amines (used in the manufacture of synthetic dyes) cause cancer of the bladder. Radium and mesothorium radioactive elements produce sarcoma of bone. Finally, benzene and the previously mentioned ionizing radiations can cause the malignant disease of the blood-forming tissues (spleen, lymph nodes, bone marrow) which is called leukemia. All the causes of cancer that are listed here are well-demonstrated and widely accepted causes encountered in specific occupations. Many other causes are suspected on the basis of statistical and experimental research. And these are being scrutinized day by day. One point should be remembered: the agents, in general, mentioned as causing occupational cancer are hazardous in the form and in the amount in which they are handled in manufacturing processes.

**Question:** Is cancer contagious? Is it possible to catch the disease from a friend living in the same neighborhood who one comes into contact with quite often?

**Answer:** The belief that cancer is contagious—that one can "catch it" from a cancer patient—is about as old as the "cancer house" superstition—and just about as baseless. The "cancer house" superstition is that it occurs with regularity among the dwellers in certain houses. This is an old and foolish superstition.

As one disease after another was proved to be caused by a germ, it did appear likely, or at least possible, that a germ would be found for cancer, too. But this has not been the case. After some 100 years of penetrating, patient search, the body of scientific opinion stands firmly against any such origin. There is at the moment great interest in viruses as possible causes of cancer. But even if research should establish their role as inciters of cancer, it is most unlikely that viruses will be found to function as agents of contagion as we use the term today. There are, to be sure, viruses that appear to cause contagious diseases—for example, measles and infantile paralysis. But on the strength of the accumulating evidence, the relationship between viruses and cancer, if it is found to exist at all, will probably not be a simple matter of the transmission of the agent from a sick person to a well one. It is likely that the role of viruses in the origin of human cancer, if there is such a role, will turn out to be vastly more complicated. The fact is that the evidence denies that cancer is infectious. Doctors and nurses spend lifetimes in close contact with cancer patients. And yet they are no more prone to develop cancer than any other group of people. It is estimated that in any given year not less than half a million patients are under treatment for cancer, and yet the instances in which two members of the same family are stricken at or near the same time are extremely rare, in spite of close and constant proximity. There is not on record anywhere a single instance of proven transfer of cancer from one person to another. Of course, now and then we hear of husband and wife, or two otherwise closely associated persons, who both have cancer. But, again, such coincidences are bound to occur in a disease as prevalent as cancer.

**Question:** If cancer is not thought to be contagious, can it then be inherited?

**Answer:** Another old misconception about cancer is that it is inherited. How often we hear the phrase, "It's in the family," tacked on to the announcement that so-and-so had cancer. And how many women are carrying, often secretly, a burden of fear that they must sooner or later be stricken with cancer of the breast, because their mothers were. True, the occurrence of certain kinds of cancer in specially bred strains of experimental animals does appear to be controlled by hereditary factors. And there are strains of mice in which the females, after years of selective mating, will develop cancer of the breast nine times out of ten. But human genetics is a completely haphazard affair, and the rigorous breeding rules that have produced cancerous strains of mice cannot possibly operate for human beings.

But what about the families we hear of in which cancer has appeared in several successive generations, or among several sisters and brothers? Do not such instances seem to suggest that cancer is hereditary? Many examples of this sort can undoubtedly be laid to chance. The statistical probability of cancer's appearing in several members of the same family—especially over a span of two or more generations—is great enough to explain some of them. And in forming an opinion based on reports of this kind, we must remember that the diagnosis of cancer has become widely reliable only recently. Reports of cancer from a generation ago must be regarded with caution. Yet we can say that a number of careful studies of human genetics have tended to show that hereditary influences operate, sometimes powerfully, sometimes weakly, to favor the development of certain diseases, including cancers. As we have seen, the role of heredity in cancer cannot be denied. Yet the instances where it is of critical importance seem to be few and far between. Most of what we know about cancer suggests that it results from a number of influences, some of which are known, some dimly suspected, and probably many of which are as yet unrecognized. Heredity should definitely be included among the possibilities, but its weight usually appears so slight that to worry about it would be a waste of time. So it is an error to think of cancer as being inexorably heritable or even to think of heredity as being a major influence in most cases of human cancer. And it is an error that breeds a great deal of unnecessary anguish and anxiety. What influence heredity does have may be said to be one of predisposition in the complicated mixture of cancer-causing factors, and it is probably limited to certain kinds of cancer. It is closer to the truth to think of heredity, where it is a force at all, as setting the stage for cancer, rather than being a direct cause.

**Question:** I know of the X-ray examination and of biopsy method of testing for cancer but what exactly is meant by the Pap Test and how is it used to detect possible cancers in the body?

**Answer:** This is a new technique for diagnosing cancer and the Pap Test is also known as the "smear" method. Pap Test is sometimes called a "Papanicolaou smear," after Dr. George Papanicolaou who first developed it. A little fluid obtained from certain organs is spread (smeared) on a glass slide. Then the fluid is stained with dyes and examined through a microscope. When cancer cells are present in the fluid, they can be spotted with a high degree of accuracy. The Pap Test is based on the fact that cells on the surface of an organ are constantly being shed and falling off. This is true of normal cells as well as abnormal ones. In certain locations, these cast-off cells can be scooped up in the normal fluid secretions. Since there are more or less constant structural differences between cancer cells and their normal brothers, the cancer cells can be identified. The method is rather like that of the botanist who can pick up a handful of leaves from the ground and tell what kind of tree each leaf fell from—provided the leaves are reasonably fresh. The Pap Test was first applied to the vagina. A cotton swab or small suction tube was used to get a drop or two of the mucous secretion that normally bathes the walls. This fluid contains cells shed from the vagina, from the surface of the neck of the womb and from the interior of the womb itself. As a rule, when cancer was present in any of these structures, cancer cells showed up in the vaginal smear—more often in the case of cancer of the cervix than in cancer of the body of the uterus. Then, as experience accumulated, it became apparent that cancer cells could appear in the smear even when the cancer was so small that it was invisible to the eye of the examining doctor. Here was an exciting prospect: being able to find cancer of the uterus—the leading cause of death from cancer among women—earlier than had ever been possible before. The smear technique soon was put to other uses. It was learned that cancer cells could be found in the sputum of most patients with cancer in their lungs. The urine of patients suffering from cancer in the bladder and of the kidney was found to contain cancer cells. Later, methods were devised for getting specimens for smears from the stomach, from the colon, and from the prostate. A lot of doctors do not feel that the smear provides the final diagnosis of cancer. Generally, a positive smear diagnosis furnishes strong evidence of the presence of cancer, but biopsy is still held essential for a final decision. Still the smear method has certain unique advantages. The ease and speed with which a smear can be taken from the vagina make it an ideal method for screening or testing large numbers of women for cancer of the uterus. A smear can sometimes point to the presence of cancer of the uterus before any signs or symptoms have appeared. It can do the "scouting" for the more certain biopsy, and can make diagnosis possible months before it would otherwise be made. Also, smears from organs like the lung, stomach, and kidney can provide strong evidence of cancer which is not accessible to biopsy without an operation. Smears are easy enough to get, but to examine them accurately calls for painstaking care. Sometimes when malignant cells are present they are spotted at once, but often they can be found only after persistent searching. And only after a thorough scanning of the entire smear can the examiner be sure that none are there. This is a slow process at best. For this reason, the capacity of cytology (cell study) laboratories will be limited until some faster technique is devised.

**Question:** Is there such a thing as the cancer personality? Is it possible that a person's emotional make-up could make one susceptible to the disease?

**Answer:** It is known that stress or emotion affects the nervous system which in turn affects the body's metabolism which acts on the glands in such a way as to make individual cells susceptible to the effects of a cancer-causing substance. You can see in some people prolonged and silent sorrow or hurt and frustration, without the release of sobs and tears. This might give rise to the saying: "Something's eating them up inside." Perhaps the death of a child, a spouse or another loved one plays an important part in the chain of events that results in cancer. It is an interesting theory. In different marital conditions among women it might be presumed, therefore, that there would be the largest incidence of cancer among widows, the next largest among those who have been divorced or separated, less among those who were legally married whether or not much remained of a happy relationship and least among single women. A survey of cancer statistics in 1956 showed that this was the case, where there were adequate statistics to work with. Other statistical studies seemed to show similar trends. Invariably widows in all age groups had a higher cancer mortality than happily married or single women. Psychiatrists delved deeper and found that apparently there was a relationship between incidence of cancer and unhappy relationships with other members of the family, especially, so it seems, an unresolved conflict with the mother of the family. Extensive studies have been done showing that there is apparently a very definite connection between certain kinds of personality and cancer incidence. Time and again, the "cancer personality" is described as a person who has a defensive attitude toward society, more anxieties than normal and less ability to reduce tension by some outward manifestation. That is, the person who broods silently rather than shouting when he is angry; the person who grieves and harbors silent fears and grudges, who cannot work off a feeling of depression, anger or frustration with exercise, singing, hard manual labor, or loud talking. Then too, there seemed to be a certain undoubted relationship between emotions and the state of a patient who succumbed to cancer. Without exception almost, the cancer patient reacts with certain definite emotional and also physical changes to the degree of illness or the deaths of patients around him. The need for narcotics varies, there are chemical changes in the urine and so forth. There seems to be some sort of relationship between the kind of personality one has and the time newly discovered cancer results in death. And there seems to be some connection, little understood, between the kind of personality and location of the cancer. It seems that the best idea is to do everything you can do to avoid being the kind of person who seems to be most susceptible to cancer—depressed, silent, worrying, anxious, resentful or "all wrapped up in yourself." Aside from a definite conscious effort to turn one's thoughts in a happier direction, there is the necessity to do everything possible to create a body so radiantly healthy that happiness is unavoidable. We are sure that following the program of a well-balanced diet, exercise, rest and good daily habits will bring about this state of mind. Isn't this, perhaps, one of the most important steps on the road to cancer prevention?

**Question:** In attempting to remove cancer by surgery, what, if any, are the complications? It would seem to be that removal of the tumor would realistically cut off the disease, particularly in the early stages.

**Answer:** Treating cancer by surgery has only one purpose: to remove every bit of diseased tissue—down to the last lurking malignant cell. The difficulty is that the apparent or obvious tumor—what can be seen or felt—is not a safe measure of its true extent. Invisible and impalpable strands of cancer cells shade into the neighboring normal tissue, making it impossible to determine the precise extent of disease at the time of operation. Only painstaking microscopic examination of all tissue removed can provide that information. There is another difficulty in attempting to remove every bit of cancer surgically. As we know, cancer has a tendency to seed itself in tissues at some distance from the parent tumor, and this seeding, or metastasis, can occur by way of the lymph system to the adjacent lymph node depots, or by way of the bloodstream to more distant sites. Wherever the cancer cells lodge they are apt to go right on multiplying, although sometimes they remain inactive for months or years. When cancer is confined to the organ where it began, complete removal by surgery is usually possible and may reasonably be expected to result in cure. And if the cancer has spread to a regional lymph node depot, but apparently not beyond, attempts to remove all of the tissue involved can still be undertaken hopefully, although the prospects of cure are decidedly dimmer. But when cancer has breached the lymph node barrier and has become rampant, cures are rare indeed. They are not unknown, however. In actual treatment the surgeon cannot be certain of the local extent of the tumor, and cannot always be sure whether cancer has or has not spread to lymph nodes. So the safest course is to assume that the tumor does involve more tissue than it seems to and that it has spread to lymph nodes. Usually, then the surgeon's task is to remove as much of the afflicted organ as is reasonable, and to remove the lymph drainage depots along with it. This explains why most cancer operations are so radical. In some cases, when all the removed tissues are examined under the microscope, it turns out that the operation may have been larger than was necessary. Yet this is the price that must be paid for the best chance in curing all the other cases, in which the disease is more extensive than it seemed.

Two examples: Small cancers of the lip are often cured by a limited surgical removal of the involved portion of the lip, but more extensive cancers require removal of the lymph nodes of the neck as well. Cancers of the mouth tend to spread to the lymph nodes of the neck, so that nodes of the neck are often removed too. Surgery for cancer of the lung now includes the lymph nodes that lie alongside the windpipe. Running through all the above discussion is the surgical principle that underlies most operations for cancer: the tumor itself is removed together with a generous margin of apparently normal adjacent tissue and the neighboring lymph nodes. And the surgeon tries to remove all this material together, en bloc, to avoid cutting across any tissues that might possibly harbor cancer cells. The spread of cancer from its starting place to neighboring lymph nodes, then to distant and multiple sites, tends to hold true for carcinomas—the malignant tumors arising in epithelial tissue. But it is not typical of the less common sarcomas—the malignant tumors of connective or supporting tissues. Most sarcomas mestastasize, too, but they do so in a single step. Cells break away from the primary tumor and enter the bloodstream, which carries them directly to distant organs like the lungs and bones where they establish numerous colonies. This tendency makes sarcomas less curable than most carcinomas. Yet when there is no physical or X-ray evidence that metastasis has taken place, vigorous efforts to remove the tumor completely are justified. Since sarcomas commonly affect an arm or a leg, amputation is often the answer. When they arise in abdominal organs or elsewhere, the surgeon tries to remove liberal amounts of the tissue surrounding the tumor.

**Question:** In attempting to destroy cancer by irradiation, is the disease vulnerable to the action of penetrating rays some of the time or all of the time? Or is irradiation not at all effective as a treatment of cancer?

**Answer:** X-rays were discovered in 1895 and radium in 1898. Within a few short years, researchers had learned a great deal about the general effect of these agents on living tissue. And they uncovered the curious fact that X-rays and radium did more damage to cancerous tissue than to normal healthy tissue. The intricate details of the effects of these powerful radiations on living cells, especially on cancer cells, are still being studied. But one thing is clear: when cells are in the process of rearranging their internal structure to get ready for immediate cell division—mitosis—they are decidedly vulnerable to the action of penetrating rays. Amounts of radiation that have no observable effects on normal cells cause profound changes in the cells of cancer. Under certain conditions, the radiation totally destroys them.

Within a matter of hours after exposure to these rays, the malignant cells show striking changes. At first, cell division ceases rather abruptly. Somewhat later, it begins again. But now it is chaotic and incomplete. Within a week, growth activity ceases, and the cells enlarge and begin to disintegrate. Their final destruction is hastened by the arrival of squads of the body's police cells. At last, the dead malignant cells are replaced by fibroblasts—faithful units of repair that we call scar tissue. The cells of different types of cancer vary in their resistance to the damaging effects of irradiation. And the cells of even the same type of cancer in two different patients differ in their response. In general, the more rapidly growing and undifferentiated a cancer is, the harder its cells are hit by the rays. This ought to mean that the wilder tumors are more readily cured by irradiation than are the less aggressive ones. And if all other considerations were equal, this would undoubtedly be true. But there are other aspects of the variation in growth activity among tumors which usually more than cancel out the advantage of radiation-sensitivity in tumors of higher grades—the more unmanageable kind. The most important is their habit of spreading early and widely to distant parts.

The discovery that cancer cells were more vulnerable than healthy cells to X-rays and radium led to the use of these rays in treatment. Enough exposure to the rays was permitted to destroy or severely damage cancer cells. Yet, it was hoped, not enough to affect normal cells seriously. Theoretically, this principle should make it possible to cure all cancers. And at first it was hoped that it would. But soon a discouraging fact became clear: often the dose required to kill cancer also did permanent harm to the surrounding normal tissue. And this fact continues to be the major limitation in the use of X-rays and radium in treating cancer today. Still, many kinds of cancer—those that can be brought into reasonably direct contact with the rays—can be destroyed entirely. And it has been found that X-rays generated at very high voltages have less undesirable effects on normal tissues and probably will be more useful in treating certain cancers because a somewhat larger total dose can be delivered to the tumor. Recently, streams of minute electrical charges from the atom-smashing betatron have been directed at cancer in human patients. The early returns seem to show that these streams can be concentrated largely in the tumor area. Thus an even greater selective action can be exerted than has been possible with radiant energy before. It is hoped that this new technique will save lives which conventional X-rays cannot.

**Question:** How are isotopes and hormones, which I have just begun to hear about these past few years, used in the treatment of cancer?

**Answer:** There are 98 elements which occur in nature and which make up the entire fabric of our world—living and nonliving. An isotope is a twin brother to an element, looking like his brother in every way and differing only in weight. Some elements, like radium and uranium, and a number of isotopes as found in nature are unstable. They emit continuous streams of particles and rays, some of which can affect living tissue as X-rays do. Such substances are said to be radioactive, and about 40 natural isotopes have this property. Recent developments in nuclear physics have made it possible to produce in atomic ovens over 500 radioactive isotopes. But only a half dozen isotopes have so far proved useful in treating cancer. Radioactive cobalt acts on living tissue very much as radium does. Since it is cheap, large quantities of it can be assembled in one treatment unit and made to substitute for a giant radium bomb or a million-volt X-ray machine. The results are encouraging, but probably not much better than those now being obtained with super-voltage X-rays. Other radioactive isotopes are injected into the body or taken in by drinking. Their theoretical usefulness is based on certain chemical elements having affinities for certain tissues of the body—that is, they are taken up and stored in these tissues in relatively large amounts. Also, these elements occur in nature in stable form (not radioactive), but they can be made radioactive. There are two isotopes that prove particularly useful because they stay exactly where they are put, and show no fondness for any particular tissues. Gold, for one, is an element that does not enter into chemical reactions readily. So it stays put, at least in the body. Could radioactive gold be injected into and around tumors so that it would emit its tumor-damaging rays only at the site of the injection? It has been used in this way in a variety of tumors, but reasonable success has been obtained only in a few circumstances. In certain cases of cancer of the prostate, where there is no evidence of general spreading, early response suggests that the disease has been completely controlled by treatment with radioactive gold. But years must pass before we know just how effective the treatment has been. More recently, radioactive chromic phosphate, a compound as chemically inactive as gold, has been injected directly into tumor-bearing areas. The initial results have been encouraging, especially in some patients with cancer of the prostate. Both radioactive gold and radioactive chromic phosphate are proving helpful in controlling the accumulation of fluid in the abdominal chest cavity. This is a fairly frequent and distressing complication of cancer which has spread to the lung covering or to the lining of the abdomen. Formerly, this fluid had to be drained off at intervals. But now, through the use of radioactive solutions, most patients require drainage less often, some of them only very occasionally. Most recently still, another radioactive isotope—yttrium—has been found to be at least as effective—and perhaps a little more so— in curbing these accumulations of fluid. Radioactive isotopes play only a small part in the treatment of cancer, and they have not borne out the hopes that they excited at first. Yet the few things they can do, they do well—better in some ways than any other type of treatment available today. We know that hormones are in some way involved in cancer. Yet it is also possible to modify in some degree the growth of at least two kinds of cancer. One of these is cancer of the breast—the commonest major form of the disease in women. The other—cancer of the prostate—the third most frequent cancer in males. In younger women, cancer of the breast that cannot be controlled by either surgery or irradiation is frequently restrained for varying periods by eliminating the major source of female sex hormones, the ovaries. Either they are removed surgically, or their functioning cells are destroyed by X-rays. Or the hormones are suppressed by administering the male sex hormone, testosterone. Two out of three patients so treated enjoy varying degrees of relief from pain and other distressing symptoms. And in one out of three, the tumors will actually become smaller—occasionally they seem to disappear altogether. Women with spreading breast cancer who are well beyond the change of life do not usually respond to testosterone, but a fair number are helped by the female hormone, estrogen.

Hormonal control is even more effective in cancer of the prostate. Most men suffering from metastatic prostate cancer that cannot be removed by surgery show striking improvement following castration or treatment with female hormone. Usually both are recommended. Experience with this type of treatment indicates that the life of the average man with advanced cancer of the prostate can be considerably extended and made relatively comfortable. Indeed, many patients now live for years after the diagnosis of what, not many years ago, would have been termed "hopeless" cancer. To all outward appearances, they are well, and they have no complaint. They still have cancer, but its activity seems to have been brought to a halt. But attempts to control breast and prostate cancer by hormones are by no means always successful. And even when the initial results are gratifying, the tumor—sooner or later—gets out of hand again. So still more heroic efforts have to be made to deprive the tumor of the stimulating effects of hormones.

**Question:** What about restraining cancer with the use of drugs?

**Answer:** A drug that would seek out and poison cancer cells but leave normal cells undamaged would surely qualify as the long-sought cancer cure. And much research is under way to find drugs that will do just this. Researchers have come up with about 25 chemical compounds that will poison cancer cells and stop or slow their growth. But all of them damage normal cells as well, though to a lesser degree. At the present time, they cannot be used long enough or in large enough doses to kill all the cancer cells, because before that their effect on normal tissue—the blood-forming tissue, for the most part—reaches the danger point, and they must be discontinued, at least for a while. Yet we do have substances that will destroy all the cancer in experimental animals without killing the animals. So it is not unreasonable to expect that some day drugs will be developed that can be used to treat cancer in humans effectively. Even now, a few of these drugs will interrupt for varying lengths of time the course of acute leukemia, which has been impossible until now. Others cause striking, though temporary, improvement in patients with Hodgkin's disease, and, occasionally, with other kinds of malignant tumors. But treatment by means of drugs and hormones and most isotopes, for that matter, does *not* lead to cure. At present, such treatment merely prolongs life and makes advanced stages of cancer more bearable.

**Question:** What about that remaining half of all the cancer patients who can not be cured at present, regardless of when or how they are treated?

**Answer:** Not too long ago, "incurable cancer" meant a steady, inexorable decline. Waning appetite, loss of weight, progressive weakness, anemia, unrelenting pain, and other distressing symptoms were all accepted as the inevitable sequels of cancer. This attitude invited premature invalidism, withdrawal, and depression. True there is still much pessimism today, but happily there are no traces of it in the better hospitals and clinics and among the better doctors. When a cure can no longer be hoped for, the goal becomes one of conserving life, or making it comfortable, and keeping it integrated. Sympathetic and resourceful doctors continue to strive toward this goal with the same interest and the same spirit they have in the face of other illness. The wasting away that is associated in the layman's mind with cancer is no longer inevitable, although it is still a feature of some cancers of the digestive system and usually appears late in the course of most fatal cancers. If the doctor and patient's family pay persistent attention to nutrition and if the patient preserves the will to live, in most cases weight and strength can be kept on throughout most of the illness. Vitamins, adequate fluids, indulgence of the patient's food preferences, nutrition between meals, substitution of frequent smaller meals for the three big ones, and a balanced, calorie-sufficient diet, perhaps with tonics to stimulate the appetite, these are what often make the difference between a house-bound invalid and a relatively active person.

We often hear people say that it is cruel to prolong the life of the hopeless cancer patient—that the most merciful thing to do is to do nothing, and let the patient slip away without prolonging the agony. There are several good reasons why doctors are unwilling to give up the fight. In the first place, the doctor's prime responsibility is to preserve life. The law demands that he accept this responsibility, but the moral factor is even more compelling. It is not the privilege of any doctor to decide that he should shorten life. The preservation of life must be the sole principle guiding medical practice, including the treatment of the hopeless cancer patient. This principle cannot be tampered with or interpreted in terms of individual ethical standards. Secondly, for a doctor to relax in the least degree his effort to maintain life means that the question of when to stop fighting will arise to plague him every time he undertakes the care of an incurable cancer patient. If it is humane to discontinue measures to prolong life by a day or two, why is it not equally merciful to stop them a week sooner? Why not two weeks or three? Where can anyone, no matter how wise, draw the line? A third reason why the doctor should never abandon the fight: now and then, cancer, even hopelessly advanced cancer, stops growing for no apparent reason. Indeed the growth disappears or regresses, and the patient is restored to health. This extraordinary event is called "spontaneous remission." It does not happen often. And when it does, science cannot usually explain it. But the fact that it does happen occasionally provides slender legitimate hope for any cancer patient. "It could happen to him." So how can a doctor do anything but give it every chance to happen by prolonging his patient's life even from day to day. One last thing, and that is the act of euthanasia, which is much talked and written about today. Euthanasia is defined as the act or practice of painlessly putting to death persons suffering from incurable and distressing disease. While the subject is exceedingly controversial in nature, we would say that it would be justifiable in one situation only, and it arises when there is no hope of relief from agony except by massive doses of narcotics. If, under these extreme circumstances, drugs to keep the patient comfortable—usually asleep—must hasten the inevitable end, then they should be given. There is a subtle difference between prolonging life and prolonging death.

**Question:** I know that Hodgkin's disease is a tumorlike process that is a form of cancer but could you tell me more about it in regard to diagnosis, treatment, etc.?

**Answer:** Although one of the rarer forms of malignant disease, Hodgkin's disease is of special interest because it affects chiefly those on the threshold of adulthood, between the ages of 20 and 30. It is about twice as frequent in males as it is in females. Hodgkin's disease is a tumorlike process that primarily involves the lymph nodes. In their normal state, these nodes are rarely larger than a small bean. So they can barely be felt even in areas where they lie close to the skin. They are present in greatest numbers in certain well-defined locations: the sides of the neck, the armpit, the groin, the mid-chest, and behind and within the abdominal cavity. The first evidence of Hodgkin's Disease is usually an enlarged lymph node, or several of them close together. And the most common location is in one side of the neck. However, any node group may be involved, and in a fair number of patients the first signs are an abdominal tumor or enlarged nodes within the chest, which are visible in X-ray pictures. A typical feature of node enlargement due to Hodgkin's disease is that it is painless and not tender. When the enlarged nodes are not detectable, anemia, fatigue, and loss of weight may be the first symptoms. If the nodes within the chest are the first to be affected, the patient may complain of difficulty in breathing before he notices anything else. Later in the disease, the symptoms become even more varied. Itching is commonly troublesome, and sometimes occurs early. The spleen is likely to become enlarged, and so may the liver. Difficulty in breathing or swallowing appears if the nodes in the chest grow large enough to compress the air or food passages. If the enlarging nodes press on veins, so as to obstruct the flow of blood, the veins may become prominent, sometimes standing out like cords; this is seen more often in the veins of the chest and neck than elsewhere. When veins of an arm or leg are blocked by masses of nodes the entire limb may be swollen. Interference with circulation in the chest or abdomen may cause fluid to accumulate in those cavities, resulting in shortness of breath or swelling of the abdomen. Periods of fever usually occur as the disease progresses. The temperature rises and falls back to normal each day for several days or weeks. Then sometimes there is an interval of weeks or months during which it remains normal. Since the duration of Hodgkin's disease may be long or short, there is no reliable way of forecasting the length of the patient's life. Occasionally the disease assumes a headlong course, and terminates within a year. At the other extreme are the patients who live for years—15 or more—with occasional episodes of active disease brought under ready control by judicious treatment. The diagnosis of Hodgkin's disease can be made with assurance only by removing one of the enlarged nodes and examining the tissue microscopically. Even then, an occasional case proves difficult to distinguish from one of the other lyphomas or from a benign enlargement. Since few tumors are more sensitive to irradiation treatment (usually in the form of X-rays) irradiation is generally used. Occasionally, if the disease seems sharply limited to a single area, it may be treated by surgical removal of the involved nodes. Recently, as well, a newly discovered chemical compound related to the mustard gas developed for chemical warfare was found to have a depressive effect on the blood-forming tissues of the body. When it was cautiously given to patients with a variety of diseases of such tissues, it proved to be of distinct benefit to some of them. And those with Hodgkin's disease responded best of all. Although there is some uncertainty as to how long life is extended by this drug treatment, it clearly brings relief and comfort to patients who no longer can expect help from irradiation.

**Question:** I have come across the name of a Dr. Max Gerson who apparently is a controversial figure in the world of cancer and its treatments. What exactly is this man's claim to fame?

**Answer:** Max Gerson, M.D. was a German-born doctor, who discovered a dietary treatment for a skin tuberculosis, in 1929. Arriving in America in 1936, he brought with him another dietary "cure"—this time for cancer. His clinic in Nanuet, New York claimed considerable success in curing, without surgery or radiation, cancers of the skin, esophagus, liver, bone, lung, breast, stomach and brain in terminal cases given up by doctors. The clinic was in operation until 1958, the year before Dr. Gerson died of pneumonia. It had been reported that the proportion of his success with patients who had been designated as terminal cases by their family doctors or specialists, was impressive. For many of them merely to remain alive for several months was a triumph. When these same patients found themselves freed from pain and able to enjoy happy, productive lives, the only accurate description for the treatment given them was "phenomenal."

The method is simple enough. Basically, it is aimed at restoring the body's chemistry to normalcy through diet. In Dr. Gerson's words, "There is no cancer in a normal metabolism . . . the liver is the center of the restoration process in those patients who improve strikingly. If the liver is too destroyed, then the treatment cannot be effective. . . . It is generally known that in cancer, especially in advanced cases, all the various metabolic systems are impaired."

Dr. Gerson believed that the metabolism of sodium and potassium, especially, is important in treating cancer patients. "Diet and medication serve the purpose of restoring potassium and the minerals of the potassium group to the tissues until they are completely saturated, and, conversely, reconveying sodium and its group out of the cells into the circulatory fluids, the connective tissues and other tissues where they belong. The retentive surplus of sodium must be eliminated. It is only on that basis that further recovery of the organs can take place," wrote Dr. Gerson.*

To accomplish this the patient is put on a very strict diet, low in animal protein, high in vegetables and fruits. There must be no alcohol, coffee, tobacco, no refined, canned or frozen foods, no foods processed in any way at all. The patient may not have any white flour or white sugar, or anything made from them. No fats, no oils, no salt substitutes are permitted. The food the patient does eat may not be prepared in a pressure cooker or an aluminum utensil. Fresh squeezed fruit and vegetable juices, as well as raw liver juice, make up an important part of the Gerson patient's diet. Along with these, much fruit, especially apples (the berry fruits are not considered desirable) and many vegetables, particularly carrots, celery, greens and potatoes, help to fill in the diet. Oatmeal and whole rye bread are also allowed. As the patient shows improvement certain types of food are restored to the diet. Protein allowances begin after the first few weeks with cheese and fish in small amounts. Eventually a full but careful natural diet is achieved. Organically grown foods are recommended for fullest success. (When an effort is being made to eliminate poisons from the body, it hardly makes sense to introduce new ones in the form of residues of insecticides and additives in the food one eats. However the Gerson treatment claims to have had its successes even when organic food was not available.) To speed the initial cleansing of the body from its poisons, the Gerson treatment calls for frequent enemas—several a day in the beginning—until the body begins to show some effective opposition to the cancer. Along with this, thyroid, lugol solution and 10 percent potassium solution, acidol pepsin capsules, lubile capsules and a 10 percent

---

*Has Dr. Max Gerson a True Cancer Cure? by S. J. Haught.

solution of caffeine potassium citrate plus injection of vitamin B-complex and liver fill out the basic Gerson treatment.

There are many in the medical profession who termed Dr. Gerson a quack, a charlatan. This gave rise to even more considerable controversy. Dr. Gerson, a recognized medical expert in Europe with many papers on cancer published in Germany, came to the United States with much esteem. In fact, in 1946 he was invited to give testimony in Senate hearings which were aimed to continue efforts to discover means of curing and preventing cancer. It was the first time in the history of the Senate that it had honored a physician in this way. Certainly he was a man of stature in medicine. But American medicine preferred to ignore the evidence of cured cases presented in Senate hearings and illustrative literature. Although the clinic claimed to have cured patients of cancer, the extent of such claims remains unconfirmed because no one was willing to investigate. Today, the Foundation for Cancer Treatment, Inc., established by a number of grateful patients to continue the publication of his teachings, has dropped out of existence for sheer lack of interest.

It was reported that one reason Gerson met opposition had to do with his alleged unwillingness to make public his method. But from the Gerson side we hear that his attempts to be published were suppressed at every turn by the American Medical Association. No official evaluation of the Gerson treatment has ever been revealed by his medical colleagues, although Dr. Gerson submitted to five investigations of his patients and their records by the Medical Society of the County of New York. Neither Dr. Gerson, nor anyone else, has ever been able to learn the results of any of those investigations. If the results are as damning as we are led to believe, why not tell the world?* The ghost of Dr. Gerson hangs over the entire question of cancer research today. Why he was not accepted by American medicine is not known for sure. He may have made mistakes in trying to introduce his revolutionary treatment to a new country. Perhaps he unwittingly antagonized influential men. The fact that he went on radio programs and sought publicity through communications outlets might have been considered ill-advised from a professional point of view. If any one of these

---

*Has Dr. Max Gerson a True Cancer Cure?* by S. J. Haught.

brought down the wrath of organized medicine, none of them should matter now. The only question to be resolved is this: can the Gerson treatment reverse the course of cancer? Some believe yes and others say no.

**Question:** I frequently see in books or on train walls a listing of the basic warning symptoms relating to cancer. I always seem to forget some of them. What are these symptoms?

**Answer:** What you are referring to as symptoms are more commonly labeled, "Cancer's Seven Danger Signals." They read as follows:

1. Any sore that does not heal.
2. A lump or thickening in the breast or elsewhere.
3. Unusual bleeding or discharge.
4. Any change in a wart or a mole.
5. Persistent indigestion or difficulty in swallowing.
6. Persistent hoarseness or cough.
7. Any change in normal bowel habits.

At this point, and in direct reference to this question, it may be wise to point out that knowledge of the Danger Signals is not enough. Although they are the earliest signs of cancer that you yourself can recognize, and although they often appear while the disease is small, localized, and highly curable, they do not necessarily appear early in the course of a cancer's growth. Some cancers can be detected by a doctor's thorough examination before they have had a chance to sound the alarm and signal their presence to you. Sometimes it is possible to find cancer in persons who seem to be perfectly well. Form the habit of having routine physical examinations periodically—not less than once a year. And in between, all men over 45 should have regular X-ray examinations of the chest, and all women over 35 should have regular vaginal smears taken. These examinations will check up on the most common areas of cancer growth. And fortunately they are simple and effective.

**Question:** I understand that bone sarcoma is a very rare kind of cancer. Yet a little girl in the neighborhood has this dread disease. Can you tell me more about it?

**Answer:** Compared with other kinds of cancer, sarcoma of the bone is rather rare. Yet it is one of the commoner tumors in children and young adults. It is found more often between the ages of five and 25 than at any other time of life.

The bones consist of connective tissue, rather than epithelial tissue that makes up the skin, the lining of the internal organs, and the various glands of the body. Malignant tumors that arise in any part of the skeleton are known as sarcomas. There are some half-dozen well-defined varieties of bone sarcoma. Each shows distinctive cellular features; each has some preference for certain sites of certain bones; each favors general age groups; and each differs somewhat from the others in respect to life expectancy and curability. To attempt to distinguish clearly among them here would be hopelessly confusing. So we shall describe them as though they were one disease, which, in a practical sense, they are. To the patient, the signs and symptoms of the various bone sarcomas do not differ appreciably. Almost any part of any bone in the body can be the starting point of a sarcoma, but there are certain preferred sites. These are: in the region of the knee—just above or just below the joint; in the thigh bone—its upper, lower, or mid portion; in the bone of the arm, especially the upper half; in the ribs; and in the pelvic bone. Malignant bone tumors are the major exception to the rule that pain is not an early symptom of bone sarcomas. The pain may be felt in a number of ways. It often comes and goes and sometimes it seems to be relieved by exercise. Or it may be so aggravated by vigorous motion that the patient tries to favor an arm or leg, an effort that often gives rise to a slight limp. At first, the patient may complain of pain in the bone or joint only at night. Or it may be worse at night than during the day. When it concerns young children, it is easy for a parent to regard such complaints lightly. But the parent should realistically think about taking his child to the doctor when the complaints persist beyond a week, if there is no distinct injury to provide a reasonable explanation. Even if the cause seems clear, an injury severe enough to be followed by pain for a week means that the child should be taken to the doctor anyway. The second important signal of bone sarcoma is a swelling caused by the expanding tumor. Sometimes this swelling may actually precede the onset of pain. When the part of the bone involved is close to the skin's surface, as in the knee, the swelling will be noticed earlier than when it is covered by heavy muscle layers, as in mid-thigh. In certain kinds of sarcoma, the skin overlying the tumor may feel warmer than elsewhere. It may be pinker than normal and have a dusky color. With very actively growing tumors, the veins in the adjacent skin may become prominent. It is known that most bone sarcomas do not respond well to X-ray therapy. They are usually treated by surgery when there is no evidence of spreading of the disease to distant organs. And, since so many of these bone tumors occur in extremities, amputation is often necessary. This is a bitter decision for parents to make. But the alternative—a limb or a life —leaves little room for hesitation. On the whole, the prospects for saving the life of a patient with bone sarcoma are dismal. One reason is the delay that usually precedes proper diagnosis. Some of this delay cannot be avoided. But, as with some other kinds of cancer, failure cannot be assigned wholly to delay. In many cases the spread of sarcoma from its point of origin takes place before the primary tumor makes itself known at all. Then, even the earliest possible treatment proves too late. This tendency to early metastasis springs from the tumor itself and nothing can be done about it—today. But avoidable delay is substantial and can often be reduced.

**Question:** I've read a statistic that cancer takes the lives of more children between the ages of one and 14 than any other disease. I found this fact shocking and would like to know more about it.

**Answer:** Indeed that statement is correct. Apart from accidents, cancer kills more youngsters in that age category. In a very general way, the rate of growth of cancer seems to be related to the age of the patient: the younger they are, the more rapid and ungovernable the cancer's course tends to be. But there are so many exceptions to this generalization that it is of little or no use in anticipating the outcome of any particular case. Yet it holds true often enough to make the treatment of cancer in children generally unsatisfactory. Another reason for these poor over-all results is that the kinds of cancer that affect children are usually different from the kinds to which adults are most susceptible. Unfortunately, they are more malignant. Further, the diagnosis of cancer in children is often more perplexing than it is in grown-ups. Since children's tumors are comparatively rare, they are less understood and less readily suspected than those that are so commonly met at older ages. And all that has been said about the tendency of early cancer to imitate many benign and trivial conditions applies equally well to young children. But the confusion is confounded because of the child's inability to express clearly his complaints. As a result, diagnosis is usually delayed until the tumor has become big enough to be noticed by a parent, and usually this is too late for cure.

**Sub-Question:** What types of cancer are most common in children?

**Answer:** First, there is retinal glioma, the tumor that occurs in the eye. Almost all victims are less than four years old, and many have not yet reached their second birthday. The retinal glioma appears to be a familiar disease, as there are records of its occurrence in half the members of a single household. Usually one eye is involved. But in one out of every four or five cases, both eyes are affected. The first sign is widening of the pupil in one eye, making the size of the two pupils unequal. This dilated pupil may resemble a squint. Somewhat later, the eye assumes a peculiar pearly glint. This whitish gleam is the tumor itself seen through the dilated pupil.

Tumors of the kidney are also among the most frequent of the malignant tumors seen in children. Almost all of these tumors are "Wilm's Tumor" (named after the doctor who first described them in detail). Since they consist of very young cells of different types, they are also known as "mixed" tumors. The average age, in this case, is three years old. The first sign of this disease is the presence of a tumor or mass in the abdomen or flank. As a rule, the parents notice some enlargement of the abdomen, more prominent on one side than the other. And it is usually this swelling which attracts attention and invites closer exploration. And a careful feeling of the abdomen then discloses a firm mass extending below the lowermost rib. Sometimes tiredness and weakness precede the discovery of swelling and tumor. And in a few cases there is bloody urine.

Neuroblastoma is a common abdominal tumor in children. This arises in the fibers of the sympathetic nerve structures behind the abdominal cavity along each side and in front of the spine.

Although neuroblastoma can develop as far down as the pelvic region, a common location is in the region of the kidney, especially in the adrenal gland, one of which perches on the top of each kidney like a cap. The fact that the adrenal is richly supplied with nerve fibers explains why neuroblastoma so often arises here.

**Sub-Question:** What about brain tumor in children?

**Answer:** Certain brain tumors are encountered as often in children as in adults, and one variety is seen only in children. Here are some symptoms which could indicate that the nervous system in the child is giving rise to a malignant tumor in the brain: disturbance of vision, which comes as "seeing double." Also, disturbance of motion as the muscular coordination is impaired. Disturbances referred to the digestive tract; such things as vomiting without preceding nausea may develop. Disturbances of personality or consciousness as the patient may appear less alert than usual. Epileptiform seizures are not uncommon. They may vary from momentary loss of consciousness so brief as to be barely noticed, to full-scale convulsions resembling in all respects the "fits" of epilepsy. And then again, headache may be the chief or only disturbance present. If it is anything possibly connected to a tumor of the brain, the headache will gradually come on more often, increase in severity, and persist longer. Obviously these signs and symptoms can be caused by conditions quite unrelated to a tumor of the brain. Yet the appearance of any one of them, or any combination of them, is important enough for a parent to call for an early medical examination.

BIBLIOGRAPHY

Battista, Orland Aloysius, *Toward the Conquest of Cancer,* Chilton Co.

Bircher-Benner M.D., M., *The Prevention of Incurable Disease,* James Clarke and Co. (England).

Bokmiller, Mathew, *The Principal Cause of Cancer,* Provoker Press.

Cameron M.D., Charles S. Cameron, *The Truth About Cancer,* Collier Books.

Gerson M.D., Max, *A Cancer Therapy: Result of Fifty Cases,* Dura Books.

Hoffman, Cecile Pollack, *People's Cancer Handbook,* Cancer Book House.

Huxley, Sir Julian Sorell, *Biological Aspects of Cancer,* Allen and Unwin Pub. (England).

Kelly, William Donald, *New Hope for Cancer Victims,* The Kelly Research Foundation.

Nolfi, Kirstine, *The Raw Food Treatment of Cancer and Other Diseases,* The Vegetarian Society (England).

Pelgrin, Mark D., *And a Time to Die,* Routledge and Paul Pub. (England).

Rodale, J. I. and Staff, *Cancer: Facts and Fallacies,* Rodale Books, Inc.

Rodale, J. I., *Happy People Rarely Get Cancer,* Rodale Books, Inc.

Scott, Cyril, *Victory Over Cancer,* Health Science Press.

Stefansson, Vilhajamur, *Cancer: Disease of Civilization,* Hill and Wang.

Tilden, J. H., *Tumors,* Health Research Pub.

Warmbrand, Max, *The Encyclopedia of Natural Health,* Groton Press.

————, *The Laetriles-Nitrilosides In the Prevention of Cancer,* The McNaughton Foundation.

# ASTHMA

**Question:** A close friend has had asthma attacks. He is particularly high-strung and angers easily. I've heard that there is a direct connection between personality and this disease. How true is this?

**Answer:** Your high-strung friend sounds definitely like the "type" of person who would be prone to asthma, if we are talking about the personality theory in relation to this disease. Because of its close affinity to emotional states of mind, asthma has been blamed on psychological reasons down through the years. Even medical dictionaries, of not too long ago, have been shown to define asthma as: "a paroxysmal (sudden attack) affliction of the bronchial tubes characterized by difficulty in breathing, cough and a feeling of constriction and suffocation. The disease is probably a neurosis." It has been said that asthmatics have in common a deep-seated emotional insecurity and an intense need for parental love and protection. One can see such traits more easily in children who have not as yet learned to disguise their emotions. They cling to their mothers, they are self-centered, usually of high intelligence, but often unable to perform well in school because of their continual anxiety that they may fail. The real or imagined rejection by parents is the cause of such behavior. There have been stories passed from book to book and lecture to lecture pointing up the psychological importance of asthma. The classic story of the man who suffered an allergy to roses tells how the sight of a rose would set him to coughing, sneezing and weeping—even if the rose happened to be made out of paper. And medical science contains some astounding stories of the relation of emotion to asthmatic attacks. A girl who fell two stories while she was cleaning a window had her first attack immediately after she hit the ground. And repressed sex impulses along with repressed fears or anger that cannot find their proper outlets may turn into an asthmatic attack. A feeling of depression may bring on an attack in some susceptible individuals. In others, the asthma may alternate with the depression. Although there are other causes of asthma to be discussed, this one concerning the emotional state of a person should not be overlooked.

**Question:** What exactly happens to the bronchial tubes when they are afflicted with asthma?

**Answer:** Bronchial asthma is an agonizing and often extremely serious ailment. The struggle for air and the labored breathing are highly distressing and can make the life of a person a torture. The difficulty in asthma exists because of an interference with the expulsion of the air from the lungs, and this interference usually takes place in the smaller branches of the bronchial tubes. Normally these bronchial tubes and their branches expand to permit the intake of air and contract to expel it. However, when they become inflamed and congested or go into a spasm they close up. This blocks the expulsion of air and upsets the whole mechanism of inspiration and expiration. In more advanced cases the affected branches of the bronchial tubes become thickened. The mucoid glands become enlarged and scar tissue forms. This causes a permanent narrowing of the small pipes through which air is inhaled and exhaled. The increase in the production of mucus further obstructs the opening through which air is carried in and out of the lungs. Hardened plugs of mucus often add to the difficulty. In very severe cases, or those of very long standing, the deterioration may reach a point where the bronchial tubes shrivel up and atrophy. At this point the power to function normally is severely and often permanently damaged. Then, parts of the lungs may become stretched by the air that is trapped in them. The stretching of the lungs brought on by the strain of bronchial attacks is known as bronchial emphysema. It should be pointed out that if the simple colds or other acute respiratory diseases that precede bronchial asthma were properly treated all along the lines of good health and proper recovery, the asthma would in most cases not develop; this holds true even where special hereditary weaknesses have created a predisposition to the illness.

**Question:** Please tell me more about the "low blood sugar" theory and the asthmatic condition.

**Answer:** Recent investigations and tests have shown that asthmatics have a consistently low blood sugar. And this seems particularly reasonable considering that diabetics (whose blood sugar is abnormally high) should not suffer from asthma. Asthmatics have an excessive amount of potassium in their blood. Diabetics have a low level of potassium. Asthmatics become worse when they eat excessive amounts of table salt. Diabetics can get along with less insulin when they take large amounts of salt. Asthmatic attacks are especially dreaded because they occur most frequently at night after a person has been asleep for several hours. In the early morning hours, the blood sugar level is at its lowest. Injections of glucose are sometimes given to asthmatic patients to relieve their attacks. This raises their blood sugar, relieving their attacks. But it does not permanently help the asthma, for taking more and more glucose (or any other form of sugar) eventually results in a still further lowering of the blood sugar. The drugs used for asthma, such as morphine, amytal and adrenalin all raise blood sugar levels. And this is most likely the reason for their temporary effectiveness. The answer to achieving a normal blood sugar level is to eliminate those foods which bring about a sudden, but short, rise in the blood sugar. In general, these are sugars and starches. The persistently low blood sugar which is believed to be a cause of asthma and other allergies, is called "hyper-insulinism," simply meaning, too much insulin.

**Question:** Is medication an answer to successful treatment of asthma?

**Answer:** It is known that drugs have failed in the treatment of the various degrees of asthma cases. Ephedrine, adrenalin and other similar symptom-relieving remedies used in the past, and in more recent years, cortisone, have not helped in these cases as far as correction is concerned. These remedies, in the long run, actually create a more chronic ailment and often endanger the life of the patient. Morphine, for example, one of the most effective drugs in the treatment of the various respiratory disorders such as asthma and emphysema, provides relief primarily by depressing the nervous centers, and then it can be labeled "as dangerous as it is effective" and that "the more serious the condition of the patient, the greater the danger." Since the dangers of morphine are recognized, many doctors hesitate to use it and instead turn to demerol, the barbiturates, chloral hydrate, alcohol, ether by rectum, and tranquilizers. However, while the baneful effects of these drugs are not obvious, they, too, can cause serious damage. Regarding demerol, sometimes in the course of a few hours this drug, in large doses, has produced serious respiratory depression and occasionally contributed to a fatal overcome. When used in acute attacks of short duration, caution should be observed because it can become habit forming. The use of sedatives to suppress or inhibit a cough is not advisable. Frequent coughing may be distressing and ineffective and may aggravate difficult breathing. It is basically a protective mechanism, and should not be suppressed. Antibiotics, especially penicillin, can cause severe allergic reactions and may, therefore, be very hazardous to any sufferer from asthma. Patients may also have violent allergic reactions to such simple drugs as aspirin. Cortisone and its related drugs such as hydrocortisone, corticotropin, prednisone and prednisolone are often used in this disease. They do not rectify the disease, and are not only hazardous to the body generally, but also turn the disease into a more serious state.

**Question:** A neighbor suffering from asthma recently sold his business and picked up his entire family, moving one and all to California. Is change in climate one of the very best ways in combating this disease?

**Answer:** This is a controversial subject. Many medical authorities are doubtful as to climate's being able to work the miracles often attributed to it. Yet, we hear continuously through the media of people who have, on recommendation, packed up and pursued that change of climate!

Barometric pressure is considered to be the most acute cause if one is talking about climate and its affecting asthma. A drop in barometric pressure, resulting in excessive humidity, can be injurious to the asthmatic. And many allergists consider pre-storm weather, with its marked pressure fluctuations, to be adverse to many asthmatics. This is not to say that it is a sure thing that an asthmatic will suffer from a quick pressure change—for many asthmatics are entirely independent of the barometer for their attacks—but those whose chest becomes tight and breathing labored for no apparent reason may find that they can predict distress periods by keeping an eye on the barometer. If sudden pressure changes are a bother, then perhaps the solution would be to change the locale to a place whose barometric pressure is fairly constant. A look at a good almanac should supply this information, or a request from the U.S. Weather Bureau would probably bring barometric data for any place in the world.

In the study of weather factors that affect asthma, other elements to be considered are wind, humidity, temperature and the altitude. Marked increases in humidity are bad for asthmatics (foggy atmospheres are considered almost intolerable). However, one can also suffer from a lack of humidity. In hot desert areas, many asthmatics suffer just as desperately as those in moist atmospheric regions. The reason is that the desert dusts are highly alkaline and may act as bronchial irritants, thereby causing attacks. Those asthmatics who are easy prey to temperature are legion, also. Some asthmatic victims react to heat and cold as others react to pollen or dust. (Pollen free areas are havens for asthmatics.) This does not mean that it takes a hot, hot summer day to make them wheeze or a winter's morning that makes one's breath freeze. Any definite change in temperature—so long as it is noticeable— will bring on the symptoms. Some people suffer attacks merely by walking in a cold wind. Though cold winds are most often named as dangerous, it has been noted that many asthmatics find that winds affect them if the wind comes from a certain direction! Of course, this phenomenon is partly explained by the fact that winds carry all types of potential irritants such as pollen, smoke, insects, dust particles, etc. Sunlight—plain, simple sunlight—plagues many asthma sufferers so that bright, pleasant days actually force them to remain indoors. The problem of controlling this disease totally by climate adjustment is that today there is probably no such thing as the perfect climate; for all occasions, certainly not. If you are near a big city, the airs are terribly polluted. And a small California town might bring just a little too much sunshine which, in one's particular case, may only irritate asthma. And paradoxically pollen, which causes much trouble, is less prevalent in the city than it is in the country. Perhaps, one hundred miles from the shore on an ocean liner one can breathe air practically free of pollen. This situation is rather expensive and also unrealistic for any permanent length of time. High mountain slopes and certain parts of this country such as California and Arizona are known to be almost free of pollen and this is why those states are most often publicized. You can have your home air-conditioned which will bring relief from wheezing at night. But it is certainly neither possible nor wise for anyone, adult or child, to stay all day in an air-conditioned house during the summer months when pollen is most abundant. Many suggest a change of climate totally as a last resort after patch tests and subcutaneous injections have failed to show a cause.

**Question:** What are the recommended methods to employ to free one from the asthmatic condition?

**Answer:** It appears certain that whatever the immediate cause, asthma would be eliminated or nonexistent if a healthful diet were universally observed. The first step is to place the patients on a protective health and body-building diet. Excluded are all refined and processed foods, all concentrated fat foods, all concentrated sweets, and all stimulants and irritants such as spices and condiments, coffee, tea, tobacco and alcohol. Milk and other dairy products are also excluded, until the attacks have been brought under complete control. In the beginning, these patients do best when they dispense with solid food altogether for several days. Hot vegetable broth, some of the hot herb teas such as alfa mint, sassafras, and linden flower tea flavored with lemon and honey, the juices of fully ripened oranges or grapefruit, or other fruit juices such as apple, grape, papaya, pineapple, diluted or whole, may be used, but no solid food. Following this, a diet composed primarily of raw and stewed fruits, small portions of lean proteins, and easily digestible vegetable carbohydrates is best. The patients must make sure they eat only small amounts of food at a time, chew their food well, and eat only when hungry. Furthermore, since they are usually in a greatly weakened condition, they must obtain a great deal of rest and sleep, and slow down in all their activities. These patients are usually highly emotional, and a change of pace toward more leisureliness and a greater degree of peace is essential. They must learn to talk slowly, to think more slowly, to breathe deeply, and to get themselves under control when tense or worried. This will not only help them to obtain better control of their emotions and modify the spasms that play a part in bringing on an attack, but will also add to their enjoyment of life. Hot baths to promote more thorough skin and kidney elimination, and enemas if necessary to maintain adequate and thorough bowel elimination, as well as a regulated program of modern physical exercises, are of great help in these cases. It should be evident that, to obtain gratifying results, this program cannot be applied haphazardly. Skillful and experienced guidance is necessary and this is why, whenever possible, the patients should be under the care of a doctor or practitioner who specializes in this type of case.

## BIBLIOGRAPHY

Davis, Adelle, *Let's Get Well,* Harcourt Brace and World.

Dublin, Louis Israel, *Mortality of Risks with Asthma,* Association of Life Insurance Medical Directors Pub.

Flatto, Edwin, *The Restoration of Health—Nature's Way,* Pyramid Books.

Davy, William Frederick, *The Physiology of the Carbohydrates,* London J. and A. Churchill.

Picker, Lorraine, *My Inward Journey,* Westminster Press.

Salter, H. H., *On Asthma—The Pathology and Treatment,* Blanchard and Lea.

# ALCOHOLISM

**Question:** If a young person finds himself liking alcohol and its effects very much, is that any indication that he must watch himself closely or fear becoming an alcoholic?

**Answer:** No individual person can be sure, in advance, that he does not have the potentiality of becoming an alcoholic. Any young person who finds himself liking alcohol or its effects, or who has any tendency to become intoxicated, should be on his guard at all times. Because alcoholism is such a devastating disease, people young and old should be educated in the direction of its avoidance.

Many opinions stress that the disease of alcoholism is essentially a disease of one's appetite and thus a nutritional disorder. If the body is seeking and enjoying alcoholic stimulation it may well be as a substitute hunger, being stimulated by the lack of proper dietary necessities. Certainly to continue to nurse the desire for alcohol can only lead in dangerous directions.

The person whose nutritional needs are high is vulnerable—he should be especially careful to avoid alcohol. Once he starts to drink, for social or other reasons, the deficiency is made worse because the alcohol crowds out of the diet the nutritious foods he should have, actually diluting the diet. So his deficiency grows worse and as it grows worse his craving for alcohol is increased, because the deficiency has somehow disrupted his appetite mechanism so that he craves the very thing that is worst for him. No one can say, therefore, that someone is an alcoholic because he simply won't "pull himself together" and stop drinking. He can't stop, any more than he can live without water or air. He has a definite physiological appetite for alcohol created by deficiency in his diet. It is not right to say that by seeing that such a person has "a good, all-around diet" he can be cured of his disease. This is the diet he was eating when he became an alcoholic. If his alcoholism indicates that he has extraordinarily high requirements for vitamins and other nutriments, then he must be given far larger amounts of these than normal people. We do not know why his requirements are so high. We just know that they are.

**Question:** In trying to overcome alcoholism completely, can an occasional nip or two hurt the treatment?

**Answer:** An alcoholic who is seeking a complete cure cannot risk taking that extra drink—social drinking—without doing harm. Overcoming the nutritional deficiency will not permit the alcoholic to drink safely as it will simply keep him from craving alcohol. A diet high in protein, fresh fruits and vegetables in which refined carbohydrates (white sugar and white flour products) are sharply curtailed or forbidden and vitamin supplements are administered should help the alcoholic get on his feet. But that is accomplished only after he resigns himself that there is to be no more drinking and the disease has been given the chance to clear up. Of course, the fact that alcoholics and their families are desperate does not make them any less susceptible to human frailty than the rest of us—but rather more so. It is hard to follow the kind of diet required; it is hard to remember to take a given number of pills at every meal, without fail. Also some patients will suffer mild upsets when they begin their doses of vitamins. Apparently something about the alcoholic's body chemistry demands that they take in such large quantities of vitamins gradually. A person cannot determine his own nutritional requirements according to those of the next door neighbors, or even a close relative. Nor can one, least of all, depend on the official recommendation for the optimum amount of each vitamin that he should be getting. An alcoholic has to be treated individually. We know he is in desperate need of good and balanced nutrition, but the diet should be administered with professional guidance to do the job most effectively.

**Question:** What exactly does alcohol do in the body and why is it often compared to what it does to diabetes?

**Answer:** First, to investigate how alcohol behaves in the body and what it does and what it does not do. Alcohol is a carbohydrate—that is, it is made of carbon, hydrogen and oxygen with a certain proportion and arrangement of molecules that differentiate it from other carbohydrates. Alcohol has been compared to acting in the body the way that gasoline acts in a car engine. The gasoline is burned to provide heat and power but it contributes nothing to the maintenance and growth of the engine. Alcohol acts as a fuel, not as a food. The impression of a stimulating effect after a few drinks is the result of the temporary lift in blood sugar. But this is followed by a sharp decline if drinking is continued. A drink dilates the tiny blood vessels at the surface of the skin, bringing with the increased amount of blood a sensation of warmth. But if the skin is exposed to cold while these vessels are dilated, body heat is lost and the whole body temperature goes down. Perhaps one reason why it keeps coming back to the comparison of alcoholism with diabetes is this—diabetes is also a disease of those individuals who cannot properly metabolize carbohydrates. In the case of diabetics, not enough insulin is produced by the pancreatic gland which has this function, so the patient suffers from high blood sugar. This is why he must be given insulin to reduce his blood sugar. In the case of alcoholics, there is too much insulin rather than too little, with the result that the alcoholic has low blood sugar. Now the answer would be simple if it were possible to drain off this extra insulin, but we find it is much more complicated than that. What causes the extra insulin that causes the low blood sugar apparently rests with the function of at least two glands—the adrenals and the pituitary. In the adrenals it is the cortex (covering) of these glands that is involved. And the pituitary are the glands regulating the adrenals. Alcoholism is caused by a deficiency in the adrenal cortical hormones—those hormones whose action is antithetical to insulin. The trouble may not be in the adrenal cortical itself, but in the master gland, the pituitary, which for some reason fails to stimulate the adrenal cortical glands as it does in normal operation of the endocrine system. It is believed, moreover, that this disability of the pituitary is not caused by the alcoholism itself but antedates its development. It is known that doctors have achieved excellent results by giving injections of ACTH and cortisone to alcoholics in their very worst condition of delirium tremens or hangovers. ACTH and cortisone are the gland extracts of the adrenal glands, in which the alcoholic is deficient. These "spectacular treatments" are a great step forward, as they provide evidence in reverse for the theory that hyperinsulinism, with its chronic partial blood sugar starvation, is an essential underlying condition of alcoholism.

We can see that the answer is to give the body a diet which regulates the blood sugar so that it does not fall below safe levels. The alcohol was needed in the first place to raise the low blood sugar level which is responsible for the "jitters," the uneasiness, the lack of confidence, the restlessness of the alcoholic, which caused him to crave alcohol.

**Sub-Question:** Does the alcoholic become an alcoholic because of his low blood sugar, or did the use of alcohol bring about the low blood sugar to begin with?

**Answer:** The answer to this question seems to be, at the present, that both these suppositions are correct. That is, the individual who has a tendency towards an improper functioning of the glands that regulate blood sugar may take to alcohol because it raises his blood sugar and thus relieves his jitters and nervousness. On the other hand, an individual who begins to drink early in life simply because of the exhilarating effect of liquor may so damage the functioning of these glands (by drinking to excess) that he eventually gets a bad case of low blood sugar in which case, of course, he feels an overpowering compulsion to go on drinking to keep his blood sugar high.

**Question:** Can you give me a diet breakdown that would aid in getting the alcoholic rid of this dread disease?

**Answer:** Here is a rundown of a recommended diet. It is so good for one's health, in fact, that the whole family should be encouraged to follow it. Naturally, alcoholic beverages do not belong on a diet list for an alcoholic, but if he follows the right diet he will not even want alcoholic beverages.

On arising he should have a fruit or vegetable juice. Then for breakfast more fruit or vegetable juice and one helping of protein food such as eggs or nuts. Two hours after breakfast more vegetable or fruit juice. For lunch, meat, fish, poultry or eggs; salad of fresh raw vegetables and greens, cooked vegetables. Then three hours after lunch a high protein snack consisting of either seeds or nuts. One hour before dinner try another vegetable or fruit juice drink and for dinner vegetables, salad, meat, fish or poultry. Two or three hours after dinner he should have another protein snack.

And then every two hours until bedtime: fruit or fruit juice, nuts or other high protein food.

In discussing the above diet realize that there are certain allowable foods under the various categories and those are the only ones that should be eaten. Allowable vegetables is everything except potatoes. Allowable juice refers to any unsweetened fruit or vegetable juice, except grape juice or prune juice. Allowable beverages are weak tea or postum and allowable desserts are fruit; unsweetened gelatine; junket (made from tablets, not the mix). Absolutely avoid using sugar, honey, rice, candy, cake, pie, pastries, custards, puddings, ice cream, spaghetti, macaroni, doughnuts, pretzels, crackers and other starchy products. Lettuce, mushrooms and nuts may be taken as freely as desired.

## BIBLIOGRAPHY

Hewitt, Donald W., *Escape From Alcohol,* Mountain View-Pacific Press.

Jones, Howard, *Alcoholic Addiction,* Tavistock Pub. (England).

Morrison, A. B., *The Low Fat Way to Health and Longer Life,* Arc Books.

Pollmer, Elizabeth, *Alcoholic Personalities,* Exposition Press

Strecker, Edward Adam, *Alcohol: One Man's Meat,* Macmillan Co.

Volderg, Edward, *Recovery From Alcoholism,* H. Regnery and Co.

Weston, Drake, *Guidebook for Alcoholics; How to Succeed Without Drinking,* Exposition Press.

Whitney, Elizabeth, *The Lonely Sickness,* Beacon Press.

William, John Roger, *Alcoholism; The Nutritional Approach,* University of Texas Press.

# DIABETES

**Question:** Why is the disease, diabetes, known as a disorder of carbohydrate (starch and sugar) metabolism?

**Answer:** While we do know that diabetes is a disorder of carbohydrate (starch and sugar) metabolism it should be pointed out initially that carbohydrate metabolism is one phase only of general metabolism. Thus, to obtain the most desirable results in diabetes cases, you not only must control the carbohydrate disorder but also the general metabolism must be rebuilt. Although diabetes has, in the past, been thought to be primarily the result of a disorder of some specialized cells of the pancreas (the islands of Langerhans), it is now well known that the liver, the nervous system, and the glands of the entire endocrine system, including the thyroid, the adrenals, and the pituitary gland are also usually involved. The portion of the brain known as the hypothalamus also plays an important role in this disease. In fact, in some cases the disease may actually show up even when the pancreas is in an apparently normal condition. The pancreas may be able to secrete the insulin needed for normal carbohydrate metabolism, and yet some other factor may interfere with its complete or effective utilization. In the obese, middle-aged person, the liver may lose the power to store glycogen and this is particularly relevant here. On the other hand, the pancreas may sometimes be found to be scarred and damaged, with calcified areas that have resulted from a previous inflammatory condition, and yet no diabetes may be present. Under normal conditions, the starches and/or sugars (known as the carbohydrates) are first converted into glucose, and then carried by the bloodstream to the liver, where they are stored in the form of glycogen for future use. In diabetes, this function has become impaired, and as a result large amounts of sugar accumulate in the blood and spill over into the urine.

**Question:** What is going on in the body when symptoms and signs of diabetes begin to show up?

**Answer:** Some of the important symptoms associated with this

193

disease are excessive thirst, a ravenous appetite, the passage of large quantities of urine, frequency of urination, loss of weight or obesity, depending upon the patient's age, the extent and duration of his illness, and his general physical condition. Visual disturbances as well as disorders of the circulation, the nervous system, and the skin are some of the later metabolic disorders that may show up in this disease. It is well known that sufferers from diabetes often suffer from a number of metabolic disorders, such as hardening of the arteries, cataracts, and hemorrhages in the eyes. Arthritis and gallbladder and kidney disorders also often accompany it. Sufferers from diabetes are also easily subject to infectious diseases and are, as a rule, prone to coronary disease. Gangrene is one of the complications that often shows up in the more advanced cases. One of the points that always must be kept in mind in connection with diabetes is that an impairment in sugar metabolism leads to an impairment in fat metabolism, and this often creates a severe problem since it causes the formation of incomplete metabolic end products such as acetone and diacetic acid, which may accumulate in the blood. These metabolic end products often cause an acid intoxication and endanger the life of the patient. In diabetes there is not only a disturbance of carbohydrate metabolism but of the whole metabolism, the metabolism of protein and the metabolism of fat. Diabetes is not a disturbance of one metabolism; it is a disturbance of the whole metabolism and the whole balance of hormones. The symptoms for diabetes can come from any part of the body function.

**Question:** What vitamin intake should be particularly emphasized in the diet of the diabetes sufferer?

**Answer:** A number of authorities do recommend that diabetics get more B vitamins in their diet than normal folks get. There is evidence that diabetic patients require more of the vitamin B complex—especially thiamin, niacin, vitamin B12 and riboflavin—than do normal people. Most of the nondescript aches and pains of the diabetic are prevented to a large extent by taking brewer's yeast with every meal. Refined foods simply do not contain all the vitamins that the original food possessed. Calcium, too, it seems, is lost by the diabetic to such an extent that decalcification of bones is common in elderly diabetics; a sure thing that bone meal should be added to food supplements. Also, it should be stressed that it is likely that the diabetic's liver is functioning improperly. This will result in the patient not being able to get all of the possible vitamin A from vegetable foods like carrots that have a lot of it. In this case, of course, vitamin A should be taken in a supplement. At the onset of diabetes great thirst is a symptom. Satisfying the thirst with large quantities of water can "wash out" the B vitamins and vitamin C, both of which are soluble in water. So it seems likely that the diabetic may be short on vitamins B and C. An injection of insulin lowers the level of vitamin C in the blood and seems to redistribute it to other parts of the body. Increasing evidence is piling up indicating that vitamin deficiencies are more common in average diets than formerly supposed. Present-day milling processes with the production of highly refined flours are robbing American foods of much of the greatly needed vitamin B complex. It has been estimated that only about 9 percent of this substance derived from grain is now present, as compared to the flours of a hundred years ago. Deficiencies in the vitamin B group have been reported in diabetes even where the calorie needs were well supplied. It would appear that pellagra-like symptoms may be induced by the rapid metabolizing of carbohydrate stores. Glossitis, cheilitis, delirium and other pellagra-like symptoms seen in certain cases have been caused to subside by the administration of nicotinic acid (or niacin, one of the B vitamins.) The so-called "protective foods" such as dairy products, eggs, green vegetables and fruits, though excellent sources of minerals and certain other vitamins, cannot be taken in sufficient quantity to compensate for the low vitamin B concentration in highly refined flour. It would seem wise, therefore, especially in diabetic diets, to avoid highly milled products and in certain instances to add the vitamin B complex in the form of concentrates or food adjuncts.

**Question:** How can a diet too high in fat be a cause of diabetes?

**Answer:** Again, we commonly think of diabetes as a disease related only to the starch part of our diet. Yet diabetes specialists know fat metabolism is also disordered in the diabetic patient. In fact, a diet too high in fat may be one of the most important causes of diabetes. It is not surprising to find that diseases of the heart and arteries are common among diabetics, for these conditions have been shown to be closely related to the amount and kind of fat eaten throughout one's lifetime. Arteriosclerosis or hardening of the arteries can be expected in practically all cases of diabetes, if they live long enough. Diabetics are particularly susceptible to coronary disease (disease of the coronary artery which leads into the heart). More than half of all living diabetics will die of some disease of the blood vessels or heart caused by "occlusion," that is, blocking of an important artery, usually the heart artery. So we see that the way the body uses fat has a great deal to do with the health of diabetics and their chance for a long and useful life. Accumulations of fatty materials (chiefly cholesterol) in the blood appear to be the cause of many heart and vascular disorders. So anything which contributes to lowering the blood level of fatty materials would seem to be beneficial for the diabetic. There seems to be much hope in regard to the unsaturated fatty acids and their help to diabetics. The unsaturated fatty acids are certain fatty compounds that appear chiefly in fats of vegetable origin. We have heard about them in relation to prostate gland disorders, skin conditions, heart and artery ailments and many more. Now we find diabetics can profit greatly from the use of food products containing large amounts of these fats. Much as a diabetic may try to control the variations of his blood sugar through diet and insulin-taking in practice one cannot expect that blood-sugar control will be maintained through the years strictly enough to keep the fats always at a minimum. Experiments have been conducted with diets high in unsaturated fats—sunflower seed oil or corn oil. When these fats were substituted in exactly equal amounts (speaking in terms of calories) to match the animal fats, it was found that the blood fats were reduced to levels unobtainable with insulin and these low levels of fat in the blood were maintained even with less insulin than usually was given. It seems quite certain that too-high levels of fat in the blood can be reduced by insulin, or, equally well, by giving unsaturated fats instead of saturated fats. The object is not to add fat to the diet, but rather to substitute one kind of fat for another. The healthy person might see that his diet contains plenty of unsaturated fats as a possible help in regulating his blood sugar so that he will never risk getting diabetes. For diabetics, it seems apparent that the wisest course is to get plenty of these healthful fats in every day's diet. It might be best to start such a program by checking exactly how much fat from animal sources you are using at present, then begin to substitute vegetable fats, while at the same time you increase your intake of the foods listed above and cut down on fatty meats. Fats from fish are good sources of unsaturated fats—the kind that reduce cholesterol—so do not cut down on these. And wheat germ oil and fish liver oil contain considerable quantities of the unsaturated fats. Be sure to include them with your daily supplements.

**Question:** How did the use of insulin for diabetes treatment come into being and how successful is its use considered today?

**Answer:** The discovery of insulin was greeted in 1922 with much hope and enthusiasm. As Banting, Best and Collip gave the world their discovery of the remedy, both sufferers and doctors alike hoped at last this was the solution to the diabetic problem. Today, it is well known that the problem has been far from solved and that the most that insulin can do is to control the symptoms of the disease, while even this is often fraught with uncertainties and danger. It has now become increasingly clear that the use of insulin often converts a simple or mild type of diabetes into a more severe and chronic condition. When insulin is used in doses that lower the sugar below normal, it actually increases the severity of the disease, because it creates what can be identified as a state of chronic insulin poisoning. This happens because large doses of insulin lead to unbalancing of the delicately adjusted glandular system, particularly the pituitary gland at the base of the skull and the cortex of the adrenal gland above the kidneys. These glands work in unison, along with the insulin-secreting pancreas, to maintain the blood-sugar level on an even keel. When too much insulin is given, it leads to a lowering of the blood sugar to a level below normal. This, in turn, activates the pituitary-adrenal system to elevate the blood sugar back to normal. The person whose body is the scene of such a tug-of-war becomes a severe diabetic, a victim of a form of poisoning in which insulin, administered to reduce the blood sugar level, indirectly but inevitably raises it. Insulin has not been without its accomplishments. By controlling excess sugar in the blood, it protects against diabetic coma. On the other hand, its use must be balanced by a carefully controlled carbohydrate intake to guard against insulin shock. Insulin shock develops when the sugar in the blood is reduced to an extremely low level. When this happens, a food that will provide sugar in a quickly absorbable form—plain sugar, orange juice, or some other sweet food—is taken to raise the sugar level in the blood. The diabetic under modern treatment is not likely to die of diabetic coma. He lives for many years and then dies from what are called complications, but are really late manifestations of the upset in metabolism which is the essence of the disease.

**Sub-Question:** What about new "remedies" to displace the use insulin?

**Answer:** In the last few years several new remedies, to be taken by mouth, have been developed. Two of them, one known as tolbutamide (Orinase), and the other as chlorpropamide (Diabinese) are sulfa preparations. Another is a somewhat different chemical composition, and is known as DBI. These remedies, too, provide a certain measure of control, but have no effect as far as lasting results are concerned, and sometimes lead to serious complications.

**Question:** What is the best program of care for sufferers of diabetes?

**Answer:** The first aim in the case of a patient suffering from this disease should be to awaken the body's own metabolic powers and promote its own functioning, or at least to help it to make a good start in this direction. To accomplish this, all extraneous influences, such as insulin or any of the other drugs commonly used in this condition should, whenever possible, be discontinued. As a next step, a diet that provides all the necessary nutritional and protective elements to promote rebuilding is important. Salt as well as other condiments and all fats are to be eliminated from the diet, and neither coffee nor tea is permitted. In addition to diet, consisting of raw vegetables in salad, cottage cheese, lean meat, fish or chicken as well as lots of grapefruit and steamed vegetables, a program of general care to promote general rehabilitation is necessary. This program includes the use of hot mineral baths every night before retiring; an abundance of rest and plenty of sleep; relaxation after each meal; and a long nap every day after lunch.

Exercise should also not be overlooked. It is not necessary to join the local gym, but a good, brisk half hour walk daily is wonderful stimulation. It improves the diabetic's tolerance for carbohydrate foods and reduces the need for insulin. Exercise lowers the blood sugar level and helps many diabetics who are overweight take off some pounds. Sugar in the urine tends to occur when a person is physically inactive and subsides when he is active. Of course, in the case of underweight diabetics whose bodies have begun to waste away, diet and insulin are necessary before the patient can begin a course of exercise.

**Question:** Has there been any theory put forth connecting the conditions of weather to diabetes?

**Answer:** Diabetes is the functional breakdown of the body's combustion engine in handling and burning glucose. And the body normally depends on this combustion of glucose for about 85 percent of its heat and energy. So we find that diabetes develops with great frequency among people who move from the south to the north and it occurs most often within the first few years after the move. This has been ascribed to the vigorous stimulation of the northern storm belt. In any world survey of diabetes, it is found that practically the only places where it is frequent and serious enough to cause alarm are the stormy, cooler regions of Europe and North America. It occurs so seldom and in such a mild form in the tropical countries that very little attention is paid to it there. The excessive stimulation of the weather in those regions where diabetes is high may cause an increased desire for sweets, for quick added energy. Also, in the regions where diabetes prevails standards of living are high, so that this desire may be satisfied to the full. In many of these regions too, less hard physical work is done, and the sugar that is eaten becomes still more excessive in terms of the body's ability to consume it. If it is at all possible, diabetics should consider moving to a warmer climate, in fact, the farther south they go, the more their symptoms are likely to abate. Going south for just the winter will also help, provided pains are taken to adjust to the northern cold on return.

BIBLIOGRAPHY

Abrahamson M.D. and Pezet, *Body, Mind and Sugar*, Holt, Rinehart, Winston.

Davis, Adelle, *Let's Eat Right to Keep Fit*, Signet Books.

Dolger and Seeman, *How to Live with Diabetes*, Pyramid Books.

Keegan, Louis, *Food Values for Calculating Diabetic and Nephritic Diets*, Macmillan Co.

Lyons, Stella, *A Diabetic's Cookbook*, A. Knopf Pub.

MacFadden, Bernarr, *Diabetes, Its Cause, Nature and Treatment*, Health Research Pub.

Pascoe, Mary, *Food for the Diabetic*, Macmillan Co.

Pavy, William Frederick, *The Physiology of the Carbohydrates*, J. and A. Churchill Pub. (England).

Pollack, Herbert, *Modern Diabetic Care*, Harcourt, Brace and Co.

# DIGESTION AND DIGESTIVE ORGANS

**Question:** I know that digestion of food starts in the mouth, but what scientifically is happening to the food in the healthy body as it is being "digested."

**Answer**: A good question as too many people take the digestive process for granted. A person puts a piece of food in his mouth, reacts to its taste and goes on to the next piece without thinking that the body is at work, intricately digesting each and every bite taken in.

The digestion of food starts in the mouth, is then continued in the stomach, and is finally completed in the small intestine. It should not be too difficult to understand why food must be eaten slowly and it must be thoroughly chewed before it is swallowed. Chewing breaks the food into small particles and mixes it with the saliva. This inaugurates the first stages of digestion, the conversion of starch into simpler forms of sugar. This change is brought about by an enzyme in the saliva called ptyalin. The saliva, which starts the digestion of the starches, is mildly alkaline.

The breakdown of food now goes into three areas of the body: stomach, small intestine, and large intestine. To answer the question in greater detail these areas will be broken up into sub-questions and answers.

**Sub-Question:** What is the stomach's function in digestion?

**Answer:** After the food has been chewed and swallowed, it enters the stomach, where the digestion of protein begins. The stomach, when empty, is a small muscular organ that can hold about 2 and a half pints of food. Its muscles are pliable, however, and it can be stretched to accommodate vastly greater amounts. The millions of glands imbedded in the walls of the stomach secrete chemical substances that start the digestion of protein, and split some of the fats into fatty acids and glycerine. Among those substances given off by the stomach glands that play an important role in stomach digestion is hydrochloric acid, which, in combination with the enzyme pepsin, starts the conversion of the various protein foods into the simpler amino acids, the building stones of the body tissues. Another enzyme, rennin, plays a special role in the digestion of the milk protein. While the ptyalin-containing saliva that starts the digestion of starch is alkaline, the gastric juice that starts the digestion of protein is normally acid. Since starches require an alkaline medium for their digestion and the stomach juices are acid in nature, starch digestion ceases in the stomach.

**Sub-Question:** What is the small intestine's function in digestion?

**Answer:** From the stomach the partly digested food is carried into the small intestine, where the last stages of digestion are completed. The small intestine is about 1 and one half inches in diameter and about 25 feet long. Its walls, like those of the stomach, contain millions of glands that secrete enzymes needed for the digestion of various food elements. These intestinal enzymes, with the aid of the bile, which is secreted by the liver, and various enzymes secreted by the pancreas and carried to the small intestine by the pancreatic duct, complete the breakup of the various elements and prepare them for absorption into the lymphatic system and the portal vein. When the food reaches the small intestine, the fat is first emulsified by the bile and then acted upon by an enzyme known as lipase, while the enzyme trypsin completes the digestion of protein, and one known as amylopsin completes the digestion of the starches. While the secretions of the stomach are of an acid nature, the secretions of the small intestine are again alkaline. It is well that these differences be kept in mind since they explain why some of the nutrition experts emphasize that concentrated starches and concentrated proteins should not be eaten together, but at separate meals. More conventional nutritionists reject this program, basing their rejection on the fact that both starches and protein are present in many foods, and that the digestive organs are usually able to handle these foods without any difficulty. What is often overlooked is the fact that foods containing both protein and starches in natural combination also possess the enzymes and other supportive elements needed for their digestion. Students of anatomy divide the small intestine, for descriptive purposes, into three sections. The upper section, the part which connects with the distal or lower end of the stomach, is the duodenum; the middle section, the jejunum; and the lower section, which connects with the large intestine, the ileum. It is important that these three divisions be kept in mind since an inflammation of ulcers in the distal or lower section of the stomach often extends into the upper section of the small intestine, the duodenum. The lower section of the small intestine, the ileum, had public attention at the time when President Eisenhower was operated upon for what is known as regional enteritis, or ileitis.

After the work of the small intestine has been completed, the digested portion of the food is picked up by countless millions of tiny velvety projections that cover the walls of the small intestine and is carried to the liver. These tiny projections, known as the villi, absorb the products of the fully digested proteins and sugars and carry them to the liver. There the proteins are further modified to make them assimilable by the cells of the body, while the sugars are stored by the liver in the form of glycogen for future use. The lymph vessels of the villi absorb the digested fat and convert it into fatty tissues to be used as padding in different parts of the body, to protect the body against injuries and insulate it against cold, and to serve as an auxiliary source of energy.

**Sub-Question:** What is the large intestine's function in digestion?

**Answer:** The food we eat contains both digestible and indigestible material. Furthermore, even digestible portions of the food are often not completely digested. The portions of the food that are indigestible or have not been completely digested are emptied into the large intestine and from there are ultimately expelled from the body. The large intestine is 5 or 6 feet long and connects with the small intestine at the lower right side of the abdomen. From there, it extends upward until it reaches the lower ribs, then crosses over to the left side, and from there turns downward again. The portion on the right side extending upward is known as the ascending colon, the portion crossing over from the right to the left side as the transverse colon, while the portion on the left side that extends downward is known as the descending colon. The part where the small and large intestines meet is shaped somewhat like a pouch, and is known as the cecum, while the end portion of the large intestine through which the undigested mass is finally expelled is known as the rectum. The undigested mass normally reaches the large intestine in a semiliquid state. This mass contains not only the indigestible portions of the food, such as fibers, cellulose etc., but also the digestible portions that have not been completely digested. There are a number of reasons why digestible portions of the food reach the large intestine undigested or only partly digested. In some cases this happens because the food has not been chewed well enough. In other cases it is because too much food has been eaten, and the digestive system could not handle all of it. At certain times, the digestive organs are overtired and cannot do a complete job. In some cases an imbalance or an insufficient supply of the digestive secretions may interfere with the digestion. The intake of foods incompatibly combined and, therefore, overtaxing to the digestive system, may also be a contributory factor.

As soon as the undigested mass reaches the upper part of the large intestine, a great deal of churning and mixing sets in. While this goes on, the fibers and other tough substances become softened and broken up. At the same time, some of the fluid is being extracted, converting the semi-liquid material into a semi-solid mass. Billions of bacteria living in the large intestine invade the fibers and the cellulose of the vegetable foods and help to disintegrate them, while the undigested or incompletely digested portion of the protein undergoes certain putrefactive changes, setting free a number of toxic by-products. These toxic by-products are often damaging to the body unless they are promptly neutralized and rendered harmless by the liver, or are counteracted by the action of other bacteria in the colon. When these changes are completed, the mass is then propelled onward by gentle wavelike contractions known as peristalsis, and is ultimately carried to the end portion of the intestine, the rectum, through which it is then expelled. The stool, when eliminated, should be well-formed of a semi-solid consistency and brownish in color. The types of food eaten influence the coloring of the stool. A preponderance of heavy proteins may cause an increase in the dark brown color; where starches, especially grain starches, predominate, the stool is often light brown, while red foods such as beets often turn the stool a dark red color. When watery, the stool has been eliminated too soon; this is diarrhea. When it is too solid, elimination has been delayed, inducing constipation. The appearance of the stool often tells an interesting story. From its content, consistency, and shape we can tell whether the bowels are functioning normally, how well the food has been digested, whether too much food has been eaten, and whether the minerals as well as the other essential nutritional elements have been fully absorbed. We can also tell whether there is bleeding in the intestinal tract; the presence of pus is an indication of tissue breakdown somewhere in the digestive tract. The amount of fat present in the feces is a key to how well the pancreas and liver are functioning. Thus, the stool may disclose a great deal about our habits and ways of living, as well as whether our digestive organs are functioning efficiently.

**Question:** What happens when the stomach becomes inflamed and is not able to function properly?

**Answer:** First, you should know that diseases of the stomach usually begin with inflammation. When the tissues of the stomach become inflamed and congested they are unable to digest food properly, and various symptoms of indigestion begin to appear. Irritating substances taken into the stomach, which the organ cannot handle, as well as toxins and irritants that circulate in the body and are carried by the bloodstream to the deeper tissues of the stomach, are often responsible for this disease. But, as well, nutritional deficiencies and nervous and emotional tensions also contribute to its development. That faulty nutrition and careless eating habits play a part in its onset should be apparent. The diet of most persons is composed of large amounts of refined and processed foods, such as white flour, processed cereals and white sugar products, and often includes excessive amounts of devitalized, concentrated foods, fried foods, coffee, tea, chocolate, liquor, artificially flavored soft drinks, and sharp spices and condiments. Furthermore, people as a rule eat too much, and too fast. They gulp their food down without chewing it, eat when not hungry, and pay very little attention to eating foods in physiologically compatible combinations. All these influences, individually and in combination, impair bodily functions, lower the resistance of the individual, and ultimately undermine the health of the digestive organs. In the early stages inflammation of the stomach (or gastritis) is usually a simple ailment and generally arises as a defense reaction on the part of the stomach tissues to irritants. It should be evident that at such time the disorder could easily be overcome, provided proper care were applied. If the ailment is neglected or improperly treated, a great deal of damage can be done. Parts of the lining and the folds of the stomach may ultimately become thickened and hardened. Polyps develop. The functioning of the secretory glands becomes progressively impaired, causing first an increase and later a decrease in the flow of gastric juices. With further damage, some parts of the lining and deeper tissues of the stomach may begin to shrink or waste away, while the secretion of the glands may diminish still further, or dry up completely. Long-standing cases of inflammation often give rise to serious malformations or lead to the development of ulcers and scars, while some cases may even break down to the point where they end with cancer. Since cases vary, it should be apparent that, whenever possible, sufferers from digestive disorders should be under the care of a competent doctor. However, to obtain results it is essential that the doctor who is in charge of the case be not only able to determine the nature of the ailment, but that he also possesses a complete understanding of how the recuperative forces of the body can be assisted to bring about recovery.

**Question:** What are the best treatments for an inflamed stomach?

**Answer:** Since we are dealing with an inflamed stomach, it should be evident that the first requirement would be to give the stomach a chance to rest and quiet down. This is why we suggest that where the vitality of the patient permits all foods should be excluded for from one to several days. Nothing but hot water flavored with a few drops of fresh fruit juice, or some of the soothing bland herbal infusions or teas should be permitted at this time. These may be taken as often as desired. An alternate program for those who are either unable or unwilling to abstain from food completely is suggested in the form of a liquid diet for several days. In the milder or earlier cases of inflammation, freshly extracted ripe grapefruit juice, whole or diluted, or, when the grapefruit juice is not well tolerated, hot freshly made vegetable broth may be used. The juice or broth may be taken about every two hours or whenever the sufferer is hungry. Use only ripe sweet grapefruits, and make sure to squeeze the juice over a glass reamer. It should be squeezed immediately before it is taken, and should be taken without sugar or any other sweetening. It should never be chilled. Apple and grape juices serve effectively, and while in season, the freshly squeezed juice of the pomegranate, whole or diluted, is an ideal drink, and the same may be said of papaya juice when obtainable. All fluids must be sipped slowly or should be taken with a spoon, a spoonful at a time. Sometimes the inflammation is of such severe nature that even the bland juice or the vegetable broth proves irritating. In these cases, a milk diet, under a doctor's care, is usually advisable at first. Only raw, skimmed milk should be used. Goat's milk, when available, is always preferable to cow's milk. Acute cases are sometimes accompanied by nausea or vomiting. In these cases, all food, even the intake of liquids, must be stopped until the nausea or vomiting is completely eliminated. Small sips of pure, cool water are sometimes tolerated, but should be used only when needed to quench thirst or relieve dryness. Sucking a lemon or lime may provide relief from nausea.

In addition to the modified fast, liquid or milk diet, other hygienic measures are usually necessary to promote elimination, induce relaxation, and promote rehabilitation and repair. Warm, cleansing enemas should be taken once daily, whenever indicated or convenient, and tolerably hot baths in which one to two glasses of epsom salts have been added to the water are recommended. Also an abundance of rest and sleep including keeping one's feet warm at all times. These measures provide the digestive organs with a chance to rest, induce relaxation, encourage elimination, and promote rehabilitation and recuperation. The fast or limited juice or milk diet is usually followed until the major symptoms have been brought under control; then a more generous diet can be instituted.

**Question:** Are there any digestive tract symptoms of vitamin deficiency and do they have any direct relation to diarrhea?

**Answer:** When you consider that every mouthful of food we eat must pass through our digestive system, you can see how important to our health is the well-being of that system. It is particularly important in the cases of vitamin deficiency. The person suffering from gastric ulcers, colitis, gall bladder trouble or any disease of the liver is much more likely to develop vitamin deficiencies, both because of the diet he may be on and because his condition prevents the body from absorbing vitamins. Various types of medication, too, are certain to result in vitamin losses. In the presence of alkalis, vitamin C, riboflavin and thiamin and perhaps even more of the vitamin B complex are destroyed in the body. This is a good reason for avoiding bicarbonate of soda or the prolonged use of any medicine that alkalizes the body. The use of several medications (magnesium trisilicate and aluminum hydroxide) for ulcers probably destroys the beneficial effects of vitamins B and C. Also the continual use of mineral oil will destroy vitamins A and D in the body. After a stomach operation, dextrose fluids are often given by injection so that the patient will not have to eat. These fluids, which are largely carbohydrates containing no vitamins at all, will deplete the body's vitamin B reserves within a few days.

Continued diarrhea will produce the same effect. This is partly because of the rapid passage of the food through the body, not leaving time for the vitamins to be absorbed and partly because the normal digestion of food may be prevented by the absence of digestive secretions. Then, too, in cases of diarrhea the processes of digestion that take place in the intestine are slowed down or eliminated entirely. Fever increases the body's metabolism, increasing its demand for vitamins. Nausea and pain incline one not to eat and again vitamin supply becomes low—at a time when there is more need for the vitamins than in a perfectly healthy state. So the whole problem becomes one of a vicious cycle in any gastrointestinal disorder. Absorption of vitamins is prevented by the disorder. Vitamin deficiency interferes with absorption even more, and so on.

**Question:** I had recently heard of the use of garlic as a remedy in curing stomach disorder. What are the pros and cons of using garlic?

**Answer:** In recent years, the question of the therapeutic value of garlic has been the object of much discussion, and the pros and cons have been more or less evenly divided.

Garlic is a bulbous plant of the lily family. It is strong-smelling and made up of small sections called cloves. The actual garlic plant has been known to be used in tablet form. The tablet could still represent the active principles of the fresh plant absorbed to vegetable charcoal, and have the advantage of being devoid of the

characteristic odor and taste. On account of the adsorptive properties of charcoal, the release of the active substances occurs gradually during the passage through the gastrointestinal tract. Any
irritative effect is thus prevented. The bactericidal action of garlic
on staphylococcus cultures (one of the most virulent of germs) was
tested and it was found that the volatile components evaporating
from freshly cut garlic exerted a considerable inhibitory action on
the growth of the bacterium. Sterile agar plates prepared with solutions of garlic remained free from growth after inoculation with
staphylococcus. Garlic is not only utilized for the treatment of
gastrointestinal infections, but has been recommended for the
treatment of various other infectious conditions. Gratifying effects
with diluted garlic juice in the treatment of purulent wounds have
been found. It is also widely recommended for the treatment of
infections of the respiratory tract. Bacteriological studies of the
feces of humans suffering from diarrhea have revealed that garlic
brings about a characteristic change in the bacterial growth. The
product has also been found to be a valuable prophylactic in
veterinary medicine.

In general, examination of the gastric juice has shown marked
increases of secretion following ingestion of garlic in patients suffering stomach disorder. This is significant as well in relation to
the aged. A large part of the beneficial results observed following
the use of garlic in chronic hypertension of the aged is due to the
intestinal putrefaction and consequent prevention of absorption of
toxic substances from the digestive tract. These patients are known
to suffer frequently from chronic constipation, intestinal obstruction or chronic appendicitis. As a result of these disorders, foodstuffs, incompletely predigested in the stomach on account of sub-
acidity or hyperacidity, reach the fecal region where they undergo
pathological putrefaction. As a consequence, toxins are absorbed
and carried into the bloodstream. This toxemia is responsible for
the varying symptoms from which these patients suffer: headache
(migraine), dizziness, fatigue, capillary spasms, etc. It is believed
that the favorable effects attributed to garlic therapy in these conditions are not due to any direct cause of dilation of the blood
vessels that the drug might effect, but to the mechanism as described above.

## BIBLIOGRAPHY

Beaumont, William, *The Experiments and Observations on the Gastric Juice and the Physiology of Digestion,* Dover Publications.

Bottomley, H. W., *Allergy: Its Treatment and Cure,* Funk and Wagnalls.

Chandler, Asa Crawford, *The Eater's Digest,* Farrar and Rinehart, Inc.

Poynter, C. W. M., *Congenital Anomalies of the Arteries and Veins of the Human Body,* University of Nebraska Press.

Rodale, J. I. and Staff, *The Complete Book of Vitamins,* Rodale Books, Inc.

Sure, Barnett, *The Vitamins In Health and Disease,* Williams and Wilkins Co.

Wattles, Wallace D., *Health Through New Thought and Fasting,* Health Research Pub.

# CONSTIPATION

**Question:** Is there more than one kind of constipation?

**Answer:** Most experts agree that there are two kinds of constipation: atonic and spastic. Atonic constipation usually affects the cecum, that is, the very beginning of the large intestine. Spastic constipation usually affects the transverse or descending colon or the rectum. The name indicates the problem that is atonic constipation—the intestine has no "tone." So, like any muscle without tone, it falls down on the job, which in this case is propelling food residues through the excretory tract. In spastic constipation the bowel is spastic—that is, it contracts in a spasm so that food residue does not pass along as it should.

**Question:** Please relate to me the causes of constipation as this condition, over the past few years, seems to be a frequently recurring source of discomfort for me.

**Answer:** First, there is the cause related to habit. One of the factors assisting defecation is the passage of 24 hours of time. You should establish the habit of defecating at a certain time of day. This is valuable as it gives the bowels a steady routine of cleansing. Posture is especially important. Since we walk upright we are inclined to have more trouble with posture than the animals who walk on all four feet. And slumping results in crowded organs and pressure on the intestines. The gastro-colic reflex is the scientific name for the "call of nature." This reflex works when food is taken which causes the bowels to begin their work of pushing the residual mass along. There is a time lag in the working of this reflex so there may be no urge to defecate for a half hour to an hour after food is taken. But it should normally occur. And if it is ignored, the reflex is weakened and gradually ceases to function as it should. Fatigue may also be a cause of constipation. Some people wake in the morning, listless and lazy, with a minimum of energy, felt throughout their entire system affecting the large intestine and the rectum. Along with this psychological state comes the emotions which when under stress can result in constipation. Two and one half to three pints of fluid a day are recommended to keep this disorder at a distance. Rest and exercise are important. For those who suffer from atonic constipation, exercise is essential, particularly walking, horseback riding, dancing—some form of rhythmic exercise. In cases of spastic constipation, just plain rest is most essential.

Some experts are particularly high on the psychic factors relating to constipation and a rooting to early childhood toilet training. The initial psychic factors refer to the hurry, nervousness, and worry associated with one's ability to have a bowel movement and concern over the necessity of defecating every day. In toilet-training children, mothers often make such an unpleasant thing out of the daily session on the toilet that the children become unnecessarily anxious about it. Eager to please, they try hard, too hard, and failure results. Such experiences can determine the habit of a lifetime. Neurotic adults are frequently constipated for psychic reasons.

**Question:** Is constipation related to other diseases?

**Answer:** Diabetes is nearly always accompanied by constipation. Individuals who have thyroid trouble suffer from constipation. It is common in obesity and almost as common among those who are reducing, if they have reduced so greatly the bulk of their meals that there is not enough to push the undigested residue through the elimination tract. Epilepsy breeds constipation and gallbladder difficulties are often accompanied by this disorder, due to overeating which has affected the gallbladder. A large percentage of stomach ulcer patients are constipated. Much constipation among ulcer patients is caused by the very treatment of the latter disease. Ulcer patients would receive a diet low in residue, and accompanied by antacid drugs to reduce the acid in their stomachs. This causes even more constipation. The relationship between these various conditions and constipation is not a causal one. It doesn't seem that constipation is necessarily responsible for other conditions. Rather, it seems, that the same things are causing both constipation and the diabetes, ulcers, epilepsy and so forth. If you rearrange your diet and your life to eliminate constipation, it seems to have a very good chance of preventing the more serious disorder.

**Question:** Is there any recommended vitamin intake with which to combat constipation?

**Answer:** Only healthy intestines are capable of doing a proper job of working the food we eat thoroughly and at a proper rate. To keep the intestines healthy, one must eat all of the necessary food elements. Vitamins are necessary in the body's proper use of proteins, carbohydrates and fats. Inositol and niacin, two of the B vitamins, prevent constipation in animals. Laboratory volunteers on diets short in thiamin, another B vitamin, become constipated. If one does not get enough B vitamins, the body simply cannot handle the carbohydrates and fats one eats. Vitamin K is another food element that is necessary in the prevention of constipation; calcium, phosphorus and other minerals must be included in the diet, too. If you wish to be certain that any one part of your body is healthy, you must make every effort to see that all parts of the body are well-nourished. Stay with a simple diet of unprocessed fresh foods, avoid white flour products and sugar and salt. On a diet such as this you'll never know what constipation is.

**Question:** I find myself an easy target for constipation. Are there any specific exercises or routines I can adhere to, for more regular and comfortable bowel movements?

**Answer:** For people, such as yourself, suffering from constipation there can be some relief through the use of exercises which are calculated to put tone into the muscles which assist in eliminating bodily waste. These muscles are especially apt to grow lazy when the individual leads a sedentary life, lacks regular exercise or is obese. Normally there is a regular activity in the muscles of the stomach and intestines which pushes food and waste through the body at a proper rate. If the muscles lag in their job and are sluggish, constipation is often the result. For a specific exercise try perching on a surface high enough above the floor to allow the feet to dangle freely. Let yourself go completely limp—head hanging on the chest, arms hanging loosely at the sides. Then straighten up—shoulders back, chest out, head far back and back arched, the arms extended to the sides. Hold this position a short time, then repeat the whole procedure about 10 times or until tired. For leg-swinging, stand on one leg, swing the other far out and far back. Change legs every 2 or 3 minutes. Individual swinging of the arms is good exercise, too. Trunk-rolling is another exercise to strengthen abdominal muscles. In this the individual stands with hands on hips and rotates his torso in a circular motion without bending the knees or moving the hips. A most effective, if somewhat difficult exercise is the following: the individual lies flat on his back, his hands at his sides. Extending his hands in front of him, he raises himself to a sitting position and leans over to touch his toes, without bending his knees or pushing himself up with his hands. Also, a therapy in which one sits Indian fashion with arms folded and legs crossed, then rises to a standing position while keeping the arms folded—this is a tough, but good exercise for the abdominals. Last, a technique that is often applied in cases of constipation is the abdominal massage. It is believed that certain constant pressure on the abdomen sometimes activates the peristaltic reflex—the contractions of the intestines which move the waste matter to the rectum—and causes renewal of the desired habits of elimination. The massage, which takes about 15 minutes, is done with the hand, while the head is slightly raised and the legs slightly flexed. The massage should begin at the upper abdomen and with a slowly kneading motion should progress downward to the pubic area. One could even use a leather or felt-covered bowling ball or cannon ball for this job. Vigorous kneading should be administered to the whole of the front and sides of the abdomen. Double-handed kneadings are excellent and round out the stomach massage, an old and much-practiced aid to elimination that is infinitely preferable to the use of laxatives and drugs. With all special exercise routines said and done, one should not forget the following which can be integrated into daily life: long walks, stooping, gardening, running, skipping, bicycling, dancing and other activities that demand physical exertion. In connection with the question of constipation, it should be noted that perfectly normal bowels will rebel in spite of exercise if proper foods are not included in the diet, or if the call for elimination is neglected or postponed. Eat well at regular times. Have a regular time at toilet and don't rush. If you feel the need for a bowel movement, go and relieve yourself at once. This, along with daily exercise, will quickly lead you to untroubled regularity.

# HEMORRHOIDS

**Question:** What exactly is this uncomfortable rectal disorder known as hemorrhoids and what is its cause?

**Answer:** A hemorrhoid is a vein that has become distended and stretched thin due to strain. This vein or veins may be situated just inside or outside the rectum. They do not lie buried deep in the flesh, but are close to the surface where they can be irritated easily. These veins serve as an auxiliary pathway for the blood and are not meant for hard use. If there is heavy pressure on the abdominal cavity, the blood takes the unimpaired alternate route. This puts a heavy load of blood on the hemorrhoidal veins and these were not meant to do heavy work. If the strain lasts any length of time or if it is often repeated, the walls of these veins gradually expand until the strain is past. Soon the elasticity is gone from them and they will no longer regain their original shape. They then expand to the point at which they can be seen and felt. These veins are then extremely sensitive and can cause true misery as well as bleeding, with even the slightest strain on the abdominal muscles. Causes of hemorrhoids are, of course, any sort of straining in bowel movements, heavy lifting, cirrhosis of the liver, pregnancy and even cancer can leave hemorrhoids as its calling card. It should be explained that heavy lifting puts strain on the abdominal muscles directly affecting the back and rectal muscles. Still it is constipation that is considered the most common cause of this condition. Constipation forces a person to strain in order to cleanse the bowels. A person is constipated when a normal, easy movement does not occur even after the normal interval has passed. The desire to cleanse the bowels can result in enormous strain in a concentrated, short period, resulting in newly acquired hemorrhoids.

BIBLIOGRAPHY

Bragg, Paul, *Building Powerful Nerve Force*, Health Science Pub.

Bragg, Paul, *Toxicless Body Purification and Healing System*, Health Science Pub.

Cummings, Richard Osborn, *The American and His Food*, University of Chicago Press.

Hall, William Whitty, *Health and Disease as Affected by Constipation*, Houd and Houghton Pub.

Hornibrook, Frederick Arthur, *The Culture of the Abdomen—The Cure of Obesity and Constipation*, Doubleday, Doran and Co.

Miles, Hallie Eustace, *Health Without Meat*, Methuen and Co. (England).

Shelton, Herbert M., *Fasting Can Save Your Life*, Health Research Pub.

Rodale, J. I. and Staff, *Encyclopedia of Common Diseases*, Rodale Books, Inc.

# ULCERS

**Question:** I hear ulcers talked about, even made light of, in everyday conversation at the office. But what exactly does it mean to be walking around with an ulcer?

**Answer:** If there is a pain centering in the pit of your stomach, just below the breastbone, which recurs often, especially within one-half to four hours after a meal, with a gnawing or aching sensation, it is likely you have an ulcer. Ulcers of the stomach are known either as gastric or duodenal ulcers, depending upon where they are located. Those in the upper stomach are known as gastric ulcers, while those found in the lower portion of the stomach, and which sometimes extend into the small intestine, are known as duodenal ulcers. Basically the types are alike, but are named differently because of their specific location. Some ulcers are extremely small, even pinpoint in size, while others may be very large. Some ulcers affect only the surface tissues, while in other cases the deeper tissues of the stomach are affected. Small ulcers in close proximity to one another often coalesce and form large ulcers, and if they are not healed they ultimately penetrate into deeper tissues and then develop into a much more serious problem. Perforation may result, and the person's life may be in danger. The size of an ulcer and how far it progresses is usually controlled by the vitality and health of the tissues, and this, in turn, is determined almost entirely by our mode of living. The pains from ulcers are often quite strong. The stomach acids irritate the sore and ulcerated areas, and cause the tissues to contract or go into spasm. This produces a great deal of suffering. Frequent bland feedings, especially the use of acid-binding protein foods, often relieve these pains. This is because proteins use up the acids and relieve the irritation. This is the reason milk is suggested in these cases, also why it is suggested that it be taken at frequent intervals or whenever the pain recurs. However, as long as the inflammation persists and the irritation continues, new quantities of acid continue to be poured out by the glands of the stomach, and then the pains recur. They usually reappear about one or two hours after a meal. In ulcers of the stomach, hemorrhages are a most serious problem. Bleeding takes place when an ulcer eats into or corrodes a blood vessel; or when mucus that has plugged up pinpoint ulcers has become loosened and been washed away, laying bare a bleeding area; or when there is oozing of blood from weak or damaged tissues. Bleeding from a superficial ulcer or from a small blood vessel may cease quickly and is more frightening than dangerous. However, oozing of blood may continue from weak or damaged tissues, or bleeding may persist from denuded pinpoint ulcers, without being noticed except through an examination of the stool for what is known as occult blood. (The term occult blood usually refers to traces of blood found in the stool.) Where bleeding continues surgery may become necessary. However, there can be no guarantee that the bleeding will not return; only when the damaged tissues are rebuilt can we be certain of permanent results.

**Question:** What are the theories related to a person's acquiring an ulcer?

**Answer:** Doctors as well as laymen often blame ulcers on nervous tension, and disregard or minimize all other precipitating factors. This is as irrational as placing the blame for an increase in chronic and degenerative diseases on aging and not on our careless and haphazard mode of living, where it really belongs. Generally, to put full blame on tension or emotional stress is a gross fallacy. Rather if one is to believe that ulcers are avoidable, then it can be suggested that those who are predisposed to the development of this disease and wish to avoid it take stock of personal habits that can help it develop. A person should be aware of unnecessary worry and overtiredness. Also he should be getting enough sleep and putting enough relaxation into every day and every weekend. Eating habits should be checked. Are you choosing the right food for your digestive tract to handle? And are you indulging too much in those social poisons—tobacco and alcohol?

Now that we have looked at the ulcer theory most generally thought of and accepted by the lay public, let's look at an ulcer development theory most physiologists subscribe to: the digestive system produces strong acids and juices designed to help break down the food one eats so that its components can be used to nourish the body. The lining of the healthy stomach is marvelously resistant to these juices and is not affected by their caustic nature. In ulcer patients, this defense of the stomach's lining against stomach acids has broken down somehow, so that, even when the ulcer patient's stomach is empty of food, the digestive juices pour forth and work away at his stomach lining as though it were food. The continued irritation of this now-delicate area soon produces a sore, known by the name of ulcer. One theory has it that ulcers spring from an inborn characteristic of the tissues. It has been said that people with blood type O have a better chance of developing an ulcer than anyone else. And that persons whose relatives have an ulcer are likely to develop the same type as the relative has. The cause of ulcers has also been described as a disturbance to the nerves which control the blood supply to the stomach lining.

If the blood does not flow freely, thus interrupting the supply of nourishment which the cells of the stomach lining depend upon for their health, these cells are in a weakened condition and open to attack. This logical interpretation of the cause of the ulcers points, as do several other theories, to the need for proper nutrition throughout the body if ulcers are to be avoided. This brings us to smoking and to the drinking of coffee. Both caffeine and nicotine are known to be enemies of vitamin C, and it is this vitamin which is necessary for maintaining healthy tissue, including that which makes up the stomach lining. A peptic ulcer is a deficiency disease reflecting a relatively high intake of refined carbohydrates and inadequate amounts of all vitamins and food minerals. The ulcer patient must learn to reject non-vitamin, non-mineral foods and to use natural high-vitamin, high-mineral foods and to keep this up for life. The eating of refined foods leads to low blood sugar and this is a prevalent condition in stomach ulcer patients. Circumstances which are responsible for the low blood sugar also can cause the ulcer. Eating of the wrong foods (especially refined carbohydrates) produces an immediate level of sugar in the blood that is very high. Then the level falls and more food is needed to keep the individual going. This raises the sugar again, temporarily, but it falls down now even faster. Thus the low blood sugar condition prevalent among ulcer patients indicates that the same wrong eating caused the ulcer just as it caused the low blood sugar. The proper nutritional diet causes blood sugar to maintain a healthy balance. And, of course, keeps a person safe from the threat of stomach ulcers.

**Question:** What are prescribed treatments for an ulcer condition?

**Answer:** The care of ulcers is tied in to proper diet, although as you will see there are certain food products tied in with good nutrition which are best to be avoided at the beginning of treatment. The care of ulcers in the stomach is begun in essentially the same way as in inflammation. It is recommended that wherever possible all solid food be completely eliminated for from one to several days and that only hot water or the soothing bland herb teas such as alfalfa, sage or camomile, flavored with a teaspoon of honey, be taken whenever the patient is hungry or thirsty. These liquids dilute and wash away the excess acid in the stomach and often provide relief. However, in the more advanced cases of ulcer or where severe damage already exists, even plain hot water or the mild herb teas may cause pain. In these cases, the use of small quantities of milk is then indicated. In very severe cases the milk may at first have to be used only in very small quantities, sometimes not more than one or two ounces at a time—but that may be taken at more frequent intervals. After the symptoms have subsided and hunger begins to assert itself, the quantity of milk may be increased and/or taken at more frequent intervals. Whenever possible, only raw skimmed milk should be used. Gradually a soft, bland diet, free of roughage, is introduced. However, the foods that are used in these cases must have an alkaline base, must be easily digestible, and must provide all essential nutrient elements, such as the valuable vitamins, minerals, and digestive enzymes, as well as the easily digestible proteins and carbohydrates. While it is true that at the onset the vitamin- and mineral-rich raw fruits and vegetables may have to be omitted in most cases, it is still imperative that the diet provide at least a minimum of all essential body and health-building elements, and it is for this reason it is urged that the easily digestible stewed fruits and steamed vegetables be included in the diet. These foods plus some of the dairy products and other easily digestible protein foods, as or whole finely ground buckwheat, will provide the nourishment well as some of the whole grain foods, such as whole brown rice that is needed in these cases in a manner that can be easily handled by sufferers from this disorder. The raw fruits and vegetables are not easily tolerated during the active stages of an ulcer condition, because these foods contain a great deal of the roughage or coarse substances irritating to the inflamed or ulcerated areas of the stomach. Nonetheless, even though these valuable foods must at first be omitted, we must still make sure to use foods which provide not only the easily digestible proteins and carbohydrates but also an abundance of the valuable vitamins, minerals, and enzymes. Fruits and vegetables provide an ample supply of these essential food elements but to obtain maximum benefits we must make sure that these foods are carefully prepared. They should be steamed in their own juices and should never be fried or overcooked. Furthermore, the liquid of these foods should never be poured off. Salt or other irritating spices and condiments should never be used, even by healthy persons. A waterless steamer for the preparation of these foods is usually more suitable. It will not only preserve their natural flavors but also most of the vitamins and minerals which less careful cooking would waste or destroy.

Fried foods are definitely dangerous to ulcer patients. It is known that unsaturated fats are rich in vitamin E, but that high heat destroys the vitamin E in them. When the vitamin E level in the blood is seen to decline, the red blood corpuscles become fragile. Patients suffering from duodenal ulcers have been known to exhibit vitamin E deficiencies. Ulcer patients, as a rule, are known to lack the necessary amount of vitamin C in their systems. After the damage has been done, and the body is apparently unable to use some natural substance like a vitamin, it has been recommended to employ vitamin C injections for beneficial results. This is necessary because the original diet for the ulcer patient, bland and lacking raw fruits and vegetables, gives an unsatisfactory supply of C. And we know that this important vitamin is necessary for the sound and rapid healing of wounds, since it is necessary for the formation of intercellular material. Its deficiency has been shown to cause a marked decrease in the tensile strength of wounds. When there is inadequate formation of the intercellular material, or collagen, the cells remain immature and blood vessels do not easily penetrate the poorly developed granulation tissue. Recently, the bioflavonoids, also known as vitamin P, have been the source of encouraging news for ulcer victims. The bioflavo-noids are found in citric solids, and other foods rich in vitamin C. Tests have shown that they can be used effectively in treating ab-normal capillary fragility and capillary bleeding. This is most significant as it is known now that inflammation of the intestinal area always precedes the appearance of an ulcer, and this inflam-mation occurs when the capillaries are weakened or damaged in some way so that they cannot do their job efficiently. The lack of nourishment to the skin surface results in soreness and, finally, eruption of an ulcer. It was logical enough that the relationship between capillary fragility and ulcers would eventually lead to the employment of bioflavonoids in the treatment of ulcer cases.

# ULCERATIVE COLITIS

**Question:** I've heard of a neighbor who died of ulcerative colitis. I was slightly familiar with the disease but had no idea that it was so life-threatening. Can you give me information regarding the course that it takes in one's body?

**Answer:** Indeed, ulcerative colitis is a most dangerous and painful disease. Colitis is an inflammation of the large intestine. When the irritation which has given rise to the inflammation persists patches of the colon become deprived of their supply of oxygen, and when this happens ulcers develop. In ulcerative colitis, the bowel movements are usually painful, loose, watery and frequent: in some cases as often as 20 to 30 times a day, often with considerable amounts of pus, mucus, and blood. Recurrent cramps and severe pains in the abdomen, rapid emaciation, severe anemia and extreme debility are some of the symptoms that accompany this disease. In this disease, some ulcers may be large, while others may be very small, even pinpoint in size. Some ulcers affect only the surface tissues, while others penetrate into the deeper tissues and, as in ulcers of the stomach, may lead to perforation. When small ulcers fail to heal, they increase in size and those which are close to one another often join and form large ulcers. The walls of the colon become hardened and thickened in some areas, friable in others. Some parts may become badly damaged and undergo a great deal of degeneration, with sloughing off of tissue, while other parts may be badly inflamed but show little or no breakdown. Polyps may develop and there may be extensive scarring that will cause a considerable degree of distortion and shrinking. To relieve the anemia, blood transfusions are often recommended, and surgery is sometimes considered necessary to cut away the badly ulcerated or hardened parts of the colon. Where this type of surgery is performed, an artificial opening has to be created through which the waste from the colon can be expelled. In cases where only part of the colon is removed, the opening is produced by connecting the abdominal wall with the remaining portion of the colon. This type of operation is known as a colostomy. Where

223

the entire colon is removed, the opening is created by connecting the abdominal wall with the ileum (the lower portion of the small intestine) and this is known as an ileostomy. This disease, as a rule, takes a long time to develop and, like ulcers of the stomach, is usually the outgrowth of irritants and toxins that affect the surface as well as the deep tissues of the colon. Emotional disturbances, nutritional abuses, dietary deficiencies, and parasitic infestation are all potential contributory factors in this disease. As with ulcers of the stomach, ulcerative colitis usually starts as a simple inflammation. The early inflammatory stages are sometimes accompanied by cramps and diarrhea or a frequent desire to move the bowels. More often the colon will simply be sore and irritated and present the characteristic signs of a spastic colon. In some cases, diarrhea will alternate with constipation.

**Question:** What care and treatment is necessary to rid one of this unfortunate disease?

**Answer:** For one, total abstention from food or, where this is not feasible or desirable, abstention from solid food for a few days is a necessary beginning. Also include a few lukewarm water enemas to clean out the bowels, and plenty of sleep, rest and warmth, as these measures will provide a fine start in the care of the early or acute case of colitis. Where a liquid diet is used, apple juice or freshly prepared hot vegetable broth is to be preferred. Citrus fruit juices may be too irritating in these cases and, therefore, should be avoided. After the acute condition is brought under control, a careful program of living and sound hygienic measures must be instituted to rebuild the weakened and damaged tissues and guard against the development of the more serious type of the disease. If the disease has already reached a more advanced stage, a more intensive program is required. Our greatest difficulties, however, are where extensive ulceration exists. In such cases, we usually have a great deal of debility and weakness, and much patience is often required before the condition can be brought under control. "Fasting," or, in other words, abstention from food, is most helpful in an early or sudden attack of acute colitis. When the colon is acutely inflamed, even small portions of food may cause irritation and increase the inflammation. When we abstain from food, or omit solid foods, we give the inflamed and irritated tissues a chance to rest and heal. Besides diet other care is also essential. The warm cleansing enemas, the relaxing hot baths, an abundance of rest and sleep, as well as good hygienic nursing care, are essential. Precautions in administering these treatments should not be overlooked. The warm cleansing enemas are recommended daily during the first two or three days to make sure that any residue that has accumulated in the colon or may cling to its walls and cause irritation is totally flushed out. However, it is important that only small quantities of water be used, usually no more than about two or three glasses at a time. After that, the enemas should be discontinued or used only when needed to relieve extreme discomfort. The good question that is often brought up is: "Why are enemas needed at all in these cases since the bowels move frequently anyhow?" To answer this, it is well to bear in mind that we are dealing with a condition in which the tissues are highly irritated and inflamed, and that any fermenting or putrefying material stagnating in the colon only increases the irritation. It is best therefore that, whenever possible, the intestinal canal be washed out. Also stagnant waste matter that clings to the walls will act as an irritant and should be loosened and eliminated. However, since the tissues are inflamed and ulcerated, it is essential that the enemas be taken cautiously, and that only small quantities of water be used. And we must make sure not to exert too much force or pressure. It is well to reiterate that the enema must at all times be regarded here as an emergency measure, and must not become a habit. It is of great help when actually needed but should be discontinued as soon as the purpose for which it is used has been accomplished. The warm baths are helpful because they are relaxing and tend to relieve the recurrent spastic pains. Hot, moist compresses applied over the abdomen are also of great help for this purpose. The patient must be trained to eat slowly and to take only small quantities of food at a time. Colitis sufferers are as a rule very irritable and restless and everything must be done to induce relaxation and emotional control. When the patient grows stronger, exercises are recommended. At the beginning, only the mildest type of exercises are suggested, usually not more than a few deep breathing exercises and gentle leg movements. As strength increases, the frequency and the type of exercises should be increased, and the patient should be encouraged to get out of bed and start walking around the house. In the more aggravated cases, it may take several weeks before definite improvement is noted. However, as time goes on the pains will gradually lessen, the bowels will begin to move less frequently, the stools will become well formed, and the mucus, pus and blood in the stools will diminish and ultimately disappear. At this stage, small quantities of finely grated raw vegetables such as carrots, turnips, cucumbers, etc., as well as some of the tender fresh raw fruits may be added to the diet. Then, we slowly add other raw vegetables as soon as we find that they can be handled without discomfort.

**Question:** If milk is often recommended to treat an ulcer what is its position in the treatment of ulcerative colitis?

**Answer:** In many ways ulcerative colitis is similar to ulcers of the stomach and sufferers from this disease, as well as those who suffer from ulcers of the stomach, require a soft, bland, nonfibrous diet. There is, though, one very striking difference in the diet of these two ailments. Milk is often of great value in ulcers of the stomach; the same is not the case in ulcerative colitis. In this disease, milk in any form is usually not well tolerated and should, therefore, be excluded from the diet. It is also known that milk is a good culture medium for bacterial growth and hence not a suitable food for those who suffer from inflamed intestines.

**Question:** Is surgery to remove part or even the whole colon something advisable in dealing with ulcerative colitis?

**Answer:** We've talked about a colostomy or ileostomy as being an operation in which the colon or ileum is connected with the abdominal wall to create an artificial opening through which the waste of the body is eliminated. But where part or all of the colon is removed, this deformity remains a permanent condition, and this is a sorry state. It should be apparent that surgery does not remove the cause of the disease, and at most provides but temporary relief, leaving the patient permanently damaged. To obtain results, the causative factors must be removed and the damaged tissues must be given a chance to heal, and this can, in the vast majority of cases, be accomplished only through the use of a carefully regulated diet and sound hygienic care. Irrespective of the amount of damage, these are the only methods that can promise complete and lasting results.

**Question:** In hearing about colitis through the years, I've recently come across something known as "diverticulitis." Exactly what is that?

**Answer:** Sufferers from spastic colitis or irritated or spastic colon sometimes develop pouches or pockets in the large intestine. These pouches or pockets are known as diverticuli and the condition is known as diverticulosis. When these pouches or pockets become inflamed, the condition is known as diverticulitis. In the acute stage, this condition is marked by pain, nausea, sometimes by vomiting and fever; while the chronic stage presents the typical symptoms of a localized colitis. These cases are sometimes operated upon, but it should be evident that this procedure does not solve the problem since diverticuli often appear in great numbers and the removal of some diverticuli or the relief of one attack does not prevent a recurrence.

### BIBLIOGRAPHY

Clark, Linda, *Get Well Naturally,* Arc Books Inc.

Copper, Lenna Francis, *Nutrition in Health and Disease,* Lippincott.

Cummings, Richard Osborn, *The American and His Food,* University of Chicago Press.

Pavy, William Frederick, *The Physiology of the Carbohydrates,* J. and A. Churchill (England).

Rodale, J. I. and Staff, *The Encyclopedia of Common Diseases,* Rodale Books, Inc.

Shelton, Herbert M., *Fasting Can Save Your Life,* Health Research Pub.

Slye, Hans, *The Stress of Life,* Health Research Pub.

Warmbrand, Max, *The Encyclopedia of Natural Health,* Groton Press.

# UNDERWEIGHT

**Question:** In our society we always seem to hear so much about all the people who are too fat. Is there such a thing as being too thin?

**Answer:** Of course, it seems perfectly natural and healthy for people to be thin. But, at the same time, there is such a thing as excessive thinness which is not attractive and can produce serious ill health. Therefore, we can say there are two types of thin people. The term "sthenic" refers to the thin people that have good muscles and the average amount of endurance and stamina. They have very good resistance to disease, they are poised and emotionally stable. They have a well balanced nervous system, but their bodies somehow just don't deposit fat. If you are this kind of person, don't worry about your "underweight." You will probably live to a healthy old age untroubled by the high blood pressure and diabetes that make your stout neighbors' lives unendurable. The other kind of thin person is called "asthenic." Such a person lacks endurance, is easy prey to fatigue and diseases, is nervous and physically weak. He is not able to meet the demands made on him by society either from a physical or personality standpoint. Usually such an individual has a narrow, shallow chest, poor posture, flabby muscles and a weak digestion. Subconsciously, he fights the idea of taking more food, for he is convinced that food does not agree with him. So he continues to grow thinner. If you are an "asthenic" type of thin person, you would do well to increase your weight if you can, for obviously the body you are walking around in is badly nourished and the outcome may not be a happy one.

**Question:** Could you tell me something about nervousness and worry in relation to one's being underweight?

**Answer:** To look at the problem of underweight and the psychological aspects connected with the disorder, it would first be wise to know the two kinds of underweight and the scientific terminology. First, there is exogenous, meaning that some people are thin simply because they do not eat enough of foods which will

228

put on weight. This is an underweight that is associated with circumstances outside the body. The other kind is endogenous, which is a thinness that has nothing to do with how much food they eat, for they may have good appetites and (without gaining a single pound) may eat as much as others in their family who are overweight. This second term refers then to circumstances arising from something inside the body. It is the first kind that directly or indirectly can deal with nervousness, worry and a host of possible tensions. We might say regarding the exogenous underweight situation that the answer is simply to eat more food. But persistent worry, psychological upsets and a feeling of being unwanted or unloved can result in lack of appetite. In fact, the whole phenomenon of psychological disorders getting in the way of appetite has become so common that it has been given a medical name itself—anorexia nervosa—nervous lack of appetite. As the appetite dwindles, and the individual eats less, his stomach shrinks accordingly; he has a desire for less and less food. As his body loses nourishment, he may develop an extremely serious condition that can result in death—death from starvation actually, although there is plenty of food around him. In the case of children, it is felt that we should very early instill in them what they will and will not eat. Why let them make the choice? Do we let our children decide whether or not they wish to go to school or what time to go to bed? Good eating habits for youngsters are certainly as important as anything else. Obviously, this is a matter needing mature judgment. And the child who is allowed to have as much candy, soft drinks, chewing gum and ice cream as he wants between meals will not have any appetite for the meats, vegetables and fruits which he should be eating at his meals. Once the bad habits are formed and you try to make some changes there could be a substantial amount of anxiety and tension as the confused youngster resents replacing the old with the new. In the case of children, parents should remember that they set examples. How can the child be taught good food habits by a father who habitually gulps down a cup of coffee for breakfast, skips lunch and then finds himself too exhausted to do justice to a dinner? Or a mother who also skips breakfast and can't be bothered to make lunch because no one else is home at lunchtime?

Bringing back appetite to adults is a little harder to accomplish. And sometimes it necessitates a firm hand and as much will power as the overweight person needs to refuse food. One element that should be kept constantly in mind is that a lack of vitamins—B vitamins particularly—results in loss of appetite. Regardless of nerves, stubbornness or deep-seated psychological hatred of food, three or four weeks of brewer's yeast or desiccated liver therapy will give any thin person an appetite—it's bound to—unless there are conditions of ill health present that prevent him from absorbing the B vitamins. Of course, it should not have to be reminded that food should be attractively served to begin with, if we are to ever tempt the appetite of a thin person.

**Question:** What about the thin person who wants to gain weight, has a good enough appetite and just can't seem to put on those much needed extra pounds?

**Answer:** This question and the subsequent answer rests with the second type of underweight as described in the previous question. This is the endogenous underweight—arising from something inside the body. The individual has a good appetite, granted, and he eats as much as the average person, but he still remains scrawny and bony, in spite of everything he can do. We are talking about deterrents to food absorption in the body and can give some conditions that prevent absorption of food, which might be what is wrong with the thin person who cannot gain weight no matter how much he eats. Lack of hydrochloric acid in the stomach or the taking of alkaline medicines such as bicarbonate of soda increases the destruction of food before the body has assimilated it. And an absence of normal digestive secretions, dysentery, colitis and other diarrheal diseases; vitamin deficiencies, drugs which prevent absorption—such as mineral oil—all interfere with absorption of food. Impaired liver function, alcoholism, hypothyroidism, therapy with one or another of the sulfa drugs, or X-ray therapy, can interfere with utilization or storage of food. Let's look at a practical example of all this. Do you take mineral oil? If so, you're bound to be suffering from a shortage of all the fat-soluble vitamins—A, D, E and K—for these are dissolved and carried away in the presence of mineral oil. Do you suffer chronically· from any condition involving diarrhea? If so, perhaps a great deal of your food is excreted without being assimilated, so that no matter how much you eat your food is doing you little good. Most advice on gaining weight will tell you to avoid bulky food that is low in calories, such as salad greens. Under no circumstances would we advise cutting out raw green, leafy vegetables—you must have those. But you can cut down to, say, one salad a day, provided you get plenty of vitamins C, A and B in food supplements. That would mean taking rose hips, fish oil and brewer's yeast or desiccated liver, which are highly concentrated sources of these three vitamins.

**Sub-Question:** What about the wasting away of energy?

**Answer:** Authorities generally agree that the most common reason for underweight among people whose appetites are good is a waste of nervous and muscular energy. If they are children, they are striving to be the best student in the class. If they are adults, they are perfectionists in everything they do, driving themselves all day long, never relaxing, and too busy to waste much time sleeping. If this is your difficulty, the only way to solve it is to begin to take it easy. Don't rush. Do everything with the least possible expenditure of energy. Don't walk if you can ride. Don't stand if you can sit. Don't sit if you can lie down. The more energy you use up in everyday activities, the more fat you are burning. And if you are suffering from excessive thinness, you need your fat. You need it to pad your bones. You need it to provide support for your abdominal organs so they will not become displaced. And you need it against some possible future day when an illness may use up even more fat and energy than you expend when you are healthy.

**Question:** Would you have a general guide giving the underweight person sound advice in gaining weight in the most nutritious way possible?

**Answer:** The easiest and quickest thing to say would be to eat three nutritious meals daily and this is true, but it can be expanded upon here to give the underweight person sound advice. First and foremost, watch that diet and don't try to gain weight by stuffing yourself on desserts and candy. A diet high in protein—meat, fish, poultry, nuts and eggs—is best for you, along with plenty of vegetables and fruits, fresh and dried. Relax and stop burning up so many calories in your daily activity. Rest before and after meals if possible. Be sure that you eat three good big meals a day and have wholesome snacks between meals and at bedtime, if this does not spoil your appetite. Eat concentrated natural foods, high in calories. Remember, though, that refined foods—white breads, bakery goods and refined cereals—will do you no good and may do you considerable harm. Make certain you are getting enough vitamins and minerals by taking food supplements. Take fish liver oil for vitamin A, brewer's yeast or desiccated liver for vitamin B and rose hips for vitamin C. At one time it was advised that a person eat all kinds of starchy foods (spaghetti, macaroni, bread and butter) for gaining weight. But more recently the thinking has been that, just as high-protein diets regulate metabolism so that the fat person loses weight, so high-protein diets are valuable for gaining weight. True, the thin person need not watch his calories on foods like potatoes and butter. But he should certainly not try to put on weight by eating refined cereals, cakes, pies, etc. A diet high in protein and starchy vegetables (prepared to retain all their vitamin and mineral content) with a minimum of sweets and plenty of fruits and vegetable oils should certainly result in gaining weight.

# OVERWEIGHT

**Question:** Is it possible to lose weight without giving up some of the things I like to eat most?

**Answer:** The average person who is overweight and desires to lose pounds wants "to have his cake and eat it," so to speak. That is, he wants some sort of miracle to take place, where the weight decreases and he keeps on going about his destructive course of dieting. Perhaps a period of healthy foods will be substituted, but it is, unfortunately, only looked at as a temporary condition. The truth is, the reason for the overweight is the wrong foods. Of course, there can be other factors, but careful selection of foods is really the source of healthy body weight, and all the pills and gadgets in the world won't help a bit if one's diet is ignored. The "pain" involved is the rejection of sweets, the elimination from the diet of pastries, salt, fried foods and second helpings. These foods must be given up. They contain the very stuff the overweight is made of, so that eating them and hoping to reduce permanently and healthfully is as foolish as heaping wood on a fire and hoping that it will go out! The theory behind diet is quite simple. It is based upon the fact that food is the fuel that keeps the body working. One's body can use only so much fuel per day to perform its job, just as a furnace can burn only so much coal to perform its job of keeping a house warm. In the case of the furnace, any extra coal piled into it will simply lie there, waiting to be used. In the body, extra food that the body can't use will lie there too—in the form of fat. To avoid having any leftover fuel that will pile up uselessly and unhealthfully, one can introduce either of two effective dietary systems into his eating. He may either weigh his food exactly to the body's needs by counting calories or he may use fuel that will not be stored at all, by eating high-protein foods which will either be used by the body as they are eaten, or be thrown off as waste, should the body be so well nourished that it has no need for them. While either of these methods is worthwhile and sensible, the calorie counting has its drawbacks. Many calorie counters are of the opinion that they will lose weight and stay healthy on a 1200-calories-a-day diet even if the 1200 calories consist of two 600-calorie pieces of pie. This reasoning, of course, can only lead to a physical breakdown much more serious than overweight. The 1200 calories must be carefully calculated to give your body the nutrients it needs to operate efficiently. The foods must be packed with protein and vitamins. Worthless foods on a low-calorie diet are, for all practical purposes, suicidal. Another objection against calorie counting is the counting itself. The constant referring to a table of numbers, and the temptation to give oneself the benefit of the doubt in borderline cases, or in foods not mentioned in the list, can lead to discouragement and eventual impatience with the whole routine. We believe the best plan for reducing is simply to rid the diet forever of any foods which the body might not be able to use or throw off. Use only completely natural foods, unprocessed and untreated and prepared in the simplest way—minus salt. This leaves out all white flour and white flour products, all refined sugars and processed fats. On such a diet one can let his appetite rule him as it did early man, who ate what he wanted and could be sure his instincts would tell him when he'd had enough. There was no danger of getting fat, because one simply didn't want to eat enough of anything to do so. With this scheme, there is no need to weigh foods or consult lists. You have only to limit your choice to natural foods and you will soon revert to your proper, healthful weight.

**Question:** What about joining a health club, setting up an exercise program and taking steam baths in order to lose weight?

**Answer:** Exercise and the like can be effective if used realistically in relation to the individual's total concept of healthy living in order to take off unnecessary weight. Many people, whether at the local health club or in the privacy of their own home, have definite programs of exercise which they are convinced will keep their weight down. Well, the principle of exercising to burn up excess calories is a sound one, but it takes a tremendous amount of exercise to make a dent in an armor of fat that's been built up over the years through ruinous eating. Many pound-foolish people can consume 3,500 calories at a single meal, yet it would take a day of active outdoor life to burn that number of calories in a man. Even a six-day bicycle rider uses only 10,000 calories per day, and his is a grind of continual physical exertion over long, long periods of time. There are few of us indeed who have the stamina for the kind of exercise that will take weight off a person who won't combine regular and careful exercise with better dietary habits. Another of the "easy ways" that doesn't do much good, and can cost a lot of money, is the steam bath. After the prescribed period of "steaming," the patient rushes immediately to a scale and discovers, to his intense joy, that there is a weight loss. But he forgets to weigh himself again after he's thirstily drunk several glasses of water to relieve the dryness caused by the loss of water sweated out, and which accounted for the temporary weight loss. It's all back on him before he's had time to pay his bill and get his clothes on.

**Question:** What is the relationship between high blood pressure and overweight?

**Answer:** It is a fact that heavyweight persons average higher blood pressure than lesser weight persons. And with a decrease of blood pressure there will be achieved, very possibly, a decrease in weight. Decreases in blood pressure reading with loss of weight are less than increases with gain of weight. In other words, if you are overweight and should decide to lose weight partly to reduce your blood pressure, it won't be nearly so easy as it would have been to keep your weight normal or below normal—and your blood pressure, too. We know the general principles of how to lose weight. A diet high in protein, low in carbohydrates and fats will take off pounds. You are offered a variety of foods, following the course of a healthy, nutritious diet, and this should not be of any great hardship on a dieter. Following the proper diet, including all your food supplements as usual, you will not be cluttering up your digestive tract with refined, processed foods and you will be nourishing your body with the necessary vitamins and minerals. If you are overweight and have high blood pressure, a diet such as this is bound to take off pounds and reduce blood pressure. If you have high blood pressure and are not overweight, try the diet anyway. If disordered blood pressure is actually caused by bad eating habits, then it seems only reasonable that any disorder of blood pressure might be prevented by eating properly and healthfully.

**Question:** I know that obesity is extremely dangerous and can cause death in certain cases. Where in the body's functioning is all the excess fat causing the most harm?

**Answer:** Everyone knows in general that overweight is unhealthful. It has been called, by many physicians, America's number one health problem. Statistics are constantly being quoted by insurance companies to show that overweight individuals are more susceptible to the degenerative diseases of middle and old age. We know that overweight individuals are much more likely to die of cancer or heart trouble. And that over 45, added fat can result in one of three conditions that are considered as the leading causes of high mortality in the obese: diabetes, hypertension (high blood pressure) and atherosclerosis (hardening of the arteries). Yes, added fat can be responsible for the much greater severity of these diseases of the blood vessels. The fat body is an unhealthy one, so perhaps the same things that produce fat also produce disorders of the circulation. The heart pumps blood through the vital organs about 10 times as fast as it does through the muscles and fatty tissues. As the amount of fat in the body increases, there is an even greater decrease in the rate at which the blood moves through the body. It has been found that the amount of blood per unit of body weight is related to the sex of the individual and also to his degree of obesity. Women have less red-blood-cell volume in proportion to their weight than men. And the fatter you get, the less blood you have circulating around, in proportion to your body weight. Lean people contain about one and a half times as much blood per pound as obese people. The lesser amount of blood circulating in the heavy people creates extra demands on the heart and probably is at least partly responsible for the tendency to heart and blood vessel disorders associated with excess weight. It's easy to see that the less blood it has to work with, in proportion to body weight, the more difficulty the heart would have in getting it to circulate properly to all parts of the body.

## BIBLIOGRAPHY

Bauer, William Waldo, *Eat What You Want,* Greenberg Press.

Bourne, Geoffrey, *Biochemistry and Physiology of Nutrition,* Academic Press.

Bronson, Barnard Sawyer, *Nutrition and Food Chemistry,* J. Wiley and Sons, Inc.

Carque, Otto, *The Key to Rational Dietetics,* Health Research Pub.

Chaney, Margaret Stella, *Nutrition,* Houghton-Mifflin.

Cummings, Richard Osborn, *The American and His Food,* University of Chicago Press.

Davis, Adelle, *Let's Eat Right to Keep Fit,* Signet Books.

Davis, Adelle, *Vitality Through Planned Nutrition,* Macmillan Co.

Duncan, Garfield G., *Diseases of Metabolism,* W. B. Saunders Co.

Fredericks, Carlton and Goodman, Herman, *Low Blood Sugar and You,* Constellation-International Pub.

Sure, Barnett, *The Vitamins In Health and Disease,* Williams and Wilkins Co.

# HEADACHES

**Question:** I am a 9 to 5 businessman who frequently gets strong headaches in the early morning hours that seem to go away after lunch. Occasionally they will come back in late afternoon. I have the feeling that my lunch meal perks up my system and gets to my head. Is there any relation between the food I'm eating and my headaches?

**Answer:** There are many, many instances where headache and dizziness are caused by low blood sugar and relieved by a high protein diet. A morning headache could be related to low blood sugar if you are in the habit of eating carbohydrates for breakfast —cereals, toast, waffles, coffee. If you suffer from headaches and especially if they occur in relation to the time you eat meals, you should definitely work towards a high protein diet. Look at the following as a sort of little vicious circle working in our systems: A high carbohydrate diet requires lots of B vitamins for its proper digestion. And all B vitamins have been removed from our popular processed carbohydrates, such as breakfast cereals, white sugar and flour. Therefore that morning meal lacks the B vitamins— most responsible for your morale. The circle is completed and the lack of a solid amount of B in a diet high in refined carbohydrates can be responsible for nervous tension and hypersensitivity mani- festing themselves as headaches. Probably your lunch is giving you a boost with added nutriments, but if that heavy head returns by late afternoon, you're still not getting the right vitamin supply. What you eat most definitely has a direct relation to how your head—and entire body for that matter—is going to feel.

**Question:** Are aspirin or similar remedies from the local drug store good cure-alls for headaches?

**Answer:** It is not believed that aspirin or similar remedies cure or prevent headaches. Of course these drugs may relieve pain, but they surely do not remove the cause, and in killing the pain, they may well bring about aftereffects or other side effects that are as bad as or worse than the headaches. It is pretty generally agreed among members of the medical profession that the worst way to treat a headache is to dose yourself with the advertised headache remedies without going to a doctor or at least trying to discover what is causing the headaches. The headache remedy—if you do not know what is really wrong—as in the case of salicylic acid, which is in aspirin, may do you serious harm. And by the constant use of headache remedies, you may develop a genuine drug addiction that will be harder to cure than the headaches.

### BIBLIOGRAPHY

Davis, Adelle, *Let's Eat Right to Keep Fit,* Signet Books.

Hackett, James Dominick, *Health Maintenance in Industry,* A. W. Shaw & Co.

LaLanne, Jack, *The Jack LaLanne Way to Vibrant Good Health,* Arc Books, Inc.

Rodale, J. I. and Staff, *The Complete Book of Vitamins,* Rodale Books, Inc.

# INSOMNIA

**Question:** I have trouble falling asleep at night. Will a sleeping pill help put an end to occasional insomnia?

**Answer:** The insomniac experiences a situation where he lies down and closes his eyes, only to begin a nightly struggle to get enough sleep to keep going through the next day. He will plump up the pillow a dozen times, rearrange the covers, change his position at least that often and be exhausted, but wide awake, as the living room clock strikes three. The person who, like yourself, is having trouble sleeping usually seeks outside help. And often the outside helper will suggest the patient get instant relief by handing him an envelope of sleeping pills. This is done to speed things up, as opposed to sitting down with the insomniac to see if some facet of his surroundings or some particular occurrence in his recent past might be the cause of the insomnia. The threat to good health that is bound up in a sleep-inducing drug is apparently not considered by many doctors. They see their job as done if the patient sleeps at night. But the patient should not be satisfied with the sleeping pill remedy. The sleeping pill is not a cure, just a postponement; it may have a toxic reaction that is immediate, or side effects that sneak up with no warning. Soon the patient is sleeping only fairly well with one tablet, so the dose is possibly upped to two; eventually, three or four might be needed to knock him out for a peaceful night. And the idea of even attempting to sleep without the nightly quota gives the insomniac the squirms. Meanwhile, instead of a wide-awake day, the drugged insomniac is bleary eyed and exhausted at work. Pep and drive diminish quickly. His emotional reactions have even changed. He's cranky, disinterested, unenthusiastic; his wife gets on his nerves and he can't stand the children. Before he was unhappy for maybe two or four of the hours he should have been sleeping, now he's miserable for the 16 hours he's awake, then he slams himself into senselessness with the sleeping tablets. This is certainly not an improvement.

**Question:** If the sleeping pill is not the healthiest means of obtaining a good night's sleep, is it possible for an insomniac to "learn" to go to sleep?

**Answer:** The weapon to fight and conquer insomnia lies within each individual troubled by this condition. You can "learn" to go to sleep, just as you "learn" to play ball or to dance. It takes practice, and others can do it naturally. There are many theories on how one can go about this learning, but the central idea, no matter what the technique used, is the relaxation of tension.

It has been said that the ideal invitation to sleep is to simply do nothing. Apparently, for an insomniac, this directive is not easily accomplished. But, in reality, unless the muscles or nerves are diseased, one possesses the ability "not to do." Tossing is doing something. So is changing position or counting sheep. This doesn't mean that one can't move around in bed, for holding a set position when you are yearning to turn is just as likely to cause tension. You've got to learn to let yourself go when you lie down at bedtime. Cease doing anything about sleep or anything else—cease all activity. Anyone can learn to do this, no matter how wide-eyed an insomniac he is. The method is known as scientific relaxation. It calls for regular practice sessions aside from bedtime, of about 45 minutes each day, until you become proficient. These periods take place in a quiet room, with the student lying on his back, outstretched. He then begins to tense each group of body muscles for several minutes (the arms, legs, trunk, facial muscles, eye muscles), then relax them, consciously allowing them to grow more and more limp. Such a procedure, it is believed, teaches the subject the contrast between tension and relaxation. Once the sensation of complete relaxation is firmly embedded in the subject's mind, he need only point his consciousness in that direction and sleep will follow with ease. Many an insomniac can help himself to sleep by arranging for as many of the following as possible: a dark room, no undue noise, a hot bath before retiring (with a gentle massage if possible), a regular hour for retiring, a large bed with a good mattress, postponement of worries or fears until tomorrow, avoidance of excitement before bedtime, mild fatigue, proper ventilation and satisfaction of any hunger pangs.

**Question:** Does the kind of bed I sleep on have a substantial effect on the kind of night's sleep I will get?

**Answer:** It has been found that the harder the mattress, the better the rest. Many tense and anxious people can relax better on a hard surface. Such an unyielding support induces a sense of security and firmness, which is translated into relaxation of the muscles. Some people will use a bed board under the mattress and relish the extra support that it gives. And for even more rigid support, since the mattress with the board under it still has some "give," the idea of covering a bed board with an inch of padding is to be considered. We say this, because then with the padding the board could be put on top of the mattress, instead of under it. The result is a product with a wooden frame which fits nicely over the sides of the bed where the mattress would ordinarily have been. The padding board is a commercial item and it would be wise to check your local medical supply or department store to see if you can get one.

**Question:** What about the generally good sleeper, who begins to wake up on various occasions and has trouble falling back to sleep?

**Answer:** When this arises, the secret is not to be too harsh on yourself. Don't begin to feel tense because you are not sleeping. If you awake during the night, relax and simply let sleep overtake you once more, rather than worrying about not being able to sleep again. These periods of wakefulness and sleep vary, anyway, with the individual. For some, the waking hours last barely long enough for a shift in position; for others, it can last for a minute or 10 minutes. If you start analyzing the fact that you are awake, this kind of activity will only build up the tenseness that fights sleep.

Remember this! If you are lying in bed for a while, and you find that you're not enjoying the rest and relaxation you should and you're beginning to thrash around, get up for awhile. Read a little, glance at a book, newspaper or magazine, and then after about half an hour try again. This time you're relaxed a little more, you have some new and pleasant thoughts, you're ready to let sleep capture you.

### BIBLIOGRAPHY

Abrahamson M.D. and Pezet, *Body, Mind and Sugar,* Holt Rinehart & Winston.

Bauer, William Waldo, *Eat What You Want,* Greenberg Press.

Davis, Adelle, *Let's Eat Right to Keep Fit,* Signet Books.

Gutwirth, Dr. Samuel, *How to Sleep Well,* Vantage Press.

Roberts, Sam E., *Exhaustion—Causes and Treatment,* Rodale Books, Inc.

Shepard, John Frederick, *The Circulation of Sleep,* Macmillan Co.

Sydenstricker, Edgar, *Health and Environment,* McGraw-Hill.

# MENTAL ILLNESS

**Question:** I've heard some things about diet and the emotionally disturbed individual. Could you tell me about the validity of this nutritional approach to mental illness?

**Answer:** For many years it has been suspected that mental illness has its origins in nutritional deficiencies. While the theory was widely known, little was done to test it. Many authorities scoffed at it, as they often do when nutrition is mentioned as a treatment for disease. It's too simple. The problem of proving the value of nutrition was complicated greatly by the fact that measuring changes in mental illness, as a result of this or that treatment, is extremely difficult. Each case can be so highly individual that comparisons with other patients, not receiving the experimental treatment (controls), actually cannot give the type of scientific evidence that stands up as undeniable proof.

Still, many experts have been showing remarkable examples of the specifics of nutrition and healthy/unhealthy state of mind. The remarkable thing though is that while the vitamin approach has been applied in some cases, the more involved use on an everyday basis is not highly thought of. And still, it is not as though mental disease were being effectively dealt with through other means. The cases mount and the hospitals overflow. Tranquilizers, shock treatments, sedatives and other commonly used measures are patently ineffective in curing most cases of mental illness. To prove a point: for example, equating the mental symptoms which occur in pellagra (a classical manifestation of thiamin deficiency) with those of most psychoses. They include memory defects, disorientation and confusion. Periods of excitement, depression, mania, delirium and paranoia occur frequently. Often these mental symptoms appear before other signs of pellagra are evident. Without these other signs, an observer would certainly not differentiate between the mental response and that shown by any other patient with similar psychiatric attitudes. Thiamin lack causes such symptoms; who is to argue that the frankly mental patient, whose symptoms are the same, could not be helped by increased thiamin in the diet, or by injections of this vitamin alone or in liver extract? Paralysis agitans, a condition characterized by continual shaking of one or more extremities which become less facile in execution of everyday exercises, was another disease submitted to vitamin therapy. In this case the administration of pyridoxine to a number of patients showed a nice improvement in a relatively good percentage. Examples go on, indicating connections between nutrition and mental problems. A general outline, as submitted in a report, goes like this: A full, nutritious diet of natural, unrefined foods. No sugar, candy, jellies, white flour products, refined cereals, polished rice or alcoholic drinks. The patient gets each day citrus juices or tomato juice, milk, meat (including liver and pork muscle), eggs, butter, salad of raw vegetables and/or fruit, and salad oil. The balance of the diet is selected from vegetables, fruits and whole grain bread. Vitamins by mouth include fish liver oil containing 10,000 units of vitamin A, and a source of the entire B-complex. Also, injections of vitamin B-complex in liver extract, or as thiamin hydrochloride—10 milligrams, riboflavin—1 milligram and nicotinic acid—100 milligrams. This kind of diet approach is recommended in treating psychiatric patients to whom specific therapy is to be administered.*

**Question:** I know that the number of mentally defective children born each year is on the rise. Is there a nutritional approach that attempts to explain this birth abnormality?

**Answer:** A recognized source of the problem of mental deficiency in children's health is the poor diet of the mother-to-be. Fifty years ago processed foods were largely unknown, candy was a sometime treat, ice cream an event and soda had barely been invented. Nowadays, the child or adult who goes through a day without all of these is considered underprivileged. In all of these foods, if they may be called that, are elements which are destructive to good health. When they are included in the diet, the body cannot hope to run at its peak efficiency. They contribute almost nothing in the way of nutrients, and what is worse they squelch

---

*"Treatment of Neuropsychiatric Disorders with Vitamins," from the *Journal of the American Medical Association,* by Dr. Norman Jolliffe, M.D.

the normal appetite for healthful foods, and destroy many of the nutrients which might happen to be present in the body. Directly, or indirectly, these nutrients are involved with the development of our intelligence. Perhaps then a supplementation of the expectant mothers' diets could contribute to suppressing mental retardation. Also, as the retarded child grows, there has been shown a definite relationship existing between nutritional status of these children and their IQ's. The younger they are when good nutrition is introduced, the greater the chance for improvement. Apparently, one of the most important factors in improving the intelligence of the retarded youngster is to begin early. This means that good nutrition is important from the moment the mother becomes pregnant on through the birth and growth of the child. A good diet for the mother does not guarantee that the baby she carries will be born a genius, but it does offer the assurance that the baby will be born with its full share of native intelligence, and normal mental and physical capacity. Once the child has arrived, plenty of love, mother's milk, plenty of B complex-rich foods, bone meal for calcium, and fresh fruits and vegetables, rich in vitamin C, should be the heart of his diet. All white sugar, white flour products should be absolutely forbidden. A foundation like this will give the brain and body a chance to develop normally. No need to wonder about the mentality of a child with this kind of nutritional history.

**Question:** Can one become mentally disturbed if he has a vitamin B12 deficiency?

**Answer:** This question pertains specifically to research that has shown a relationship between mental illness and pernicious anemia, which is largely the result of a vitamin B12 shortage. Knowing this, we can think of the number of patients who have consulted doctors on mental trouble, who might have needed vitamin B12 and nothing more, yet were pronounced hopeless. The diagnosis of mental problems due to pernicious anemia is often difficult, because they may occur without the changes in the blood usually expected when anemia is present. However, there are two tests for vitamin B12 levels in the blood which are helpful in such cases, as they show consistently low values of oxygen consumption in the brain in patients with mental disturbances due to pernicious anemia, as compared to normal people and those with anemia due to blood loss. When mental symptoms occur along with the classic symptoms of pernicious anemia—weakness, sore tongue, an increase in the size of red corpuscles, absence of digestive juices in the stomach, etc., diagnosis is easy. However, these are often absent, and the mental symptoms are not consistently characteristic. They range from mild moodiness, with difficulty in concentrating and remembering, to violent maniacal behavior, severe agitation, stuporous depression and hallucinations. The common nervous symptoms of a vitamin B12 deficiency are different and not connected with the mind at all. They include "pins-and-needles" sensations, numbness, stiffness, feelings of heat and cold, local feelings of deadness, tightness and shooting pains. If any of these are present with the mental symptoms, the diagnosis is again made somewhat easier. Investigating a B12 deficiency is certainly a worthwhile avenue for the doctor confronted with a puzzling case of mental illness. Determining a vitamin B12 deficiency is not an involved procedure. Each patient can be tested for this possibility. Such testing for all nutrients should be a matter of course when any physical problem presents itself. We have mentioned that injection is used. The reason is simply that, by the time such conditions have appeared, the stomach does not contain any, or possibly enough of a certain substance which must be present to absorb vitamin B12. So vitamin B12 taken by mouth would be wasted. Injecting the vitamin into the patient's blood or muscle assures its absorption, since it does not pass through the digestive tract at all. Of course, injection of a vitamin must be done by a physician. Meanwhile to insure oneself against the ever-increasing threat of mental illness, include some food and food supplements rich in the B vitamins (including B12 naturally) such as beef liver and other organ meats, brewer's yeast and desiccated liver in your regular diet. Remember, if vitamin B12 can be used to cure mental disorders, it should also be an excellent preventive.

**Question:** I've heard so much about blood sugar, high and low, and its relationship to almost all disorders. Now can you explain blood sugar in terms of the functioning of a healthy mind?

**Answer:** It is believed that many patients who go from doctor to doctor seeking cures for nervousness, anxiety and exhaustion are suffering from low blood sugar due to poor nutrition. Instead of being told they are neurotics, they should be given a diet to overcome the low blood sugar conditions. Rapid fluctuations in blood sugar, common in a neurotic condition, often give rise to many bizarre symptoms suggesting mental problems. Therefore, the ideal circumstance would be to give the patient a test of the amount of sugar in his blood at given intervals after he has taken a dose of sugar. This is known as the "glucose tolerance test." If the test indicates low blood sugar, the patient can be cured permanently by a simple diet, no medication or other treatment being necessary.

Low blood sugar is so common because very often when one is found to have a low blood sugar condition, a family doctor will prescribe a diet high in sugar. This only makes the situation worse. Sitting down at a sugar bowl and eating by the spoonful large amounts of sugar is certainly not to be recommended. And therefore eating foods with a large sugar content is equally foolish because they only encourage the system to rapidly crave more and more sugar which rapidly gives way to an imbalance in metabolism. To metabolize this intake, the sugar carburetory of the body must be thrown wide open and the islands of Langerhans must secrete at an abnormally high speed to produce an overabundance, causing a low blood sugar state. And it is known that a calcium deficiency as well usually goes along with low blood sugar.

The tricky thing to always remember about the low blood sugar diet is that low blood sugar is caused by too much sugar in the diet. So the cure, and the preventive, is to cut out sugar and with it those starchy foods which are rapidly changed to sugar in the body.

The object of the proper nutritional regime is to prevent blood sugar starvation by keeping a trickle of usable sugars constantly going into the bloodstream. This prevents the sudden rush of an overabundance of sugar, which is what causes the trouble by stimulating the secretion of too much insulin, resulting in an almost immediate need for more sugar.

The negative mental conditions which prevail in our society can only be an additional factor in motivating people to do things apart from normal behavior, detrimental to themselves and detrimental to society as as well. Here are some symptoms found in patients suffering from low blood sugar—characteristic of persons committing crimes as well as just "unbalanced neurotics": slowing of mental processes, dullness, difficulty in making even minor decisions, depression, anxiety, irritability, tendency to be negative, also physical symptoms like double vision, dizziness, changes in voice texture, etc. The qualities of mind most easily and earliest affected are spontaneity and initiative. Difficulty in thinking may progress to a temporary arrest of thought, and abstract thought may be almost impossible. There are disorders of orientation and consciousness, there is mental and physical fatigue, apathy and indifference, irritability and aggression.

**Question:** Is low blood sugar a far more serious problem for children than it is for adults?

**Answer:** Yes, where children are concerned, it does seem that low blood sugar may be far more serious than for adults. The importance of nutrition for mental and physical functioning is much greater in children than in adults. In adults, faulty or insufficient nutrition may alter or impair specific or general mental functions and eventually cause reparable or even irreparable structural damage of the nervous system. In children, a grave additional factor is faced. The development of the brain may be retarded, stopped, altered, and thus the mental functions may become impaired in an indirect and not less serious way. Also, repeated attacks of low blood sugar may give rise to true epilepsy. The following are symptoms of low blood sugar in children: the child overeats or does not want to eat at all. Impairment of memory in the form of amnesia is one of the most common happenings in severe cases of low blood sugar. When the child states that he did not do or say a certain thing, he may actually not remember. The child may not sleep well. Nightmares, sleep-walking or even bed wetting may be symptoms. The child does not learn. Cases have been reported in which the child failed in one subject only. He may be absent minded or mischievous or cannot remember anything. Laziness may be caused by low blood sugar, with mental fatigue, dullness, indifference, lack of initiative and above all, severe inability to make decisions. The child may be neurotic, psychopathic or have criminal tendencies, anxiety, running away, aggressiveness, a blind urge to activity, destructiveness with impairment of moral sensibilities like shame.

In its simplest form it is the tendency to deny and contradict everything. It is no wonder that a considerable number of criminal and
semi-criminal acts have been observed in children having low
blood sugar, ranging from destructiveness or violation of traffic
regulations, all the way to bestiality, arson, and homicide.

**Question:** What is the connection between a functioning thyroid
gland and one's positive condition of mental health?

**Answer:** It has been shown that the hormone produced by the
thyroid gland—thyroxin—when deficient in the body can cause a
definite slowdown of physical and mental processes. Thyroxin carries iodine which is most essential to a healthy body. The symptoms of hypothyroidism (underactive thyroid gland) include defective memory, slow mentation and attacks of irritability culmi-
nating in an outburst of homicidal violence. Reading of these
symptoms could well make us wonder just how many beds in our
mental hospitals are taken by patients who need nothing more
than additional thyroxin in their diet to become as mentally normal as the rest of us. Unfortunately, many doctors fail to look for
underactive thyroid gland as a cause of the mental disturbances
exhibited by their patient. Or if they do, until recent years there
was usually a misdiagnosis of thyroid abnormalities. The decision
was usually based upon the basal metabolism rate test. Metabolism
is the name given to the process by which the body converts food
into energy. Now this test seeks to determine just what this metabolism rate is when the patient is completely at rest. Even the act
of digestion can make this reading shoot up, so it is easily seen
how the result could be inaccurate if the patient is emotionally disturbed or exhausted. For example, anxiety over some problem
may so elevate the reading that it might falsely indicate normal
thyroid function.

Recently, a new test was developed for measuring thyroid activity, and it is much more reliable. Called the protein-bound test, it
requires nothing more from the patient than that he allow a small
sample of his blood to be taken. The sample is analyzed for iodine
content, which must be sent from the thydroid, and if the amount
of iodine exceeds or falls below the established norm, there is
trouble suspected in the gland's working. The protein-bound-
iodine test is easily available to your doctor, who has only to send

a sample of blood to one of 250 medical centers and laboratories throughout the country which are equipped to make the test. The fee is no more than the fee for the basal metabolism rate test, and this new test is a lot more accurate. It would seem important that the thyroid has a sufficient supply of iodine through the diet, so that it can be released in thyroxin when needed. Sea kelp is an excellent natural source of iodine, as are all sea foods. Thyroid trouble is basically caused by use of excessive salt, aspirin, coffee, and cigarettes in the diet. These products are known to interfere with the proper functioning of the thyroid gland which is to release the proper amount of iodine, if it has been made available through the right foods. All the above mentioned products act, in excessive amounts, as strong stimulants, and all, particularly aspirin, can have an immediate antithyroid action, with hypothyroidism the result of its use. There is hope for the slightly affected and hope for those who appear to be seriously mentally ill, if the thyroid is considered when diagnosis is made. The biochemical phase of treatment for mental illness is coming into its own, and when its importance is fully appreciated, we believe we will see, for the first time, a reversal of the upward trend in the number of mental illness cases.

## BIBLIOGRAPHY

Blaine, T. R., *Mental Health Through Nutrition,* Citadel Press.

Bragg, Paul, *Building Powerful Nerve Force,* Health Service Co.

Evans, Isabelle Walsh, *Sugar, Sex and Sanity,* Carlton Press, Inc.

Gardner, George E., *The Emerging Personality,* Delacorte Press.

Glasser, William, *Reality Therapy,* Harper and Row.

Hollingshead, August deBelmont, *Social Class and Mental Illness,* Wiley Pub.

House, Samuel Daniel, *A Mental Hygiene Inventory,* Columbia University Thesis.

Rodale, J. I., *Natural Health, Sugar and the Criminal Mind,* Rodale Books, Inc.

Stern, Edith, *Mental Illness, a Guide for the Family,* Commonwealth Fund Publishers.

Van Den Haag, Ernest, *Passion and Social Constraint,* Stein and Day.

Winick, Charles E., *The New People,* Pegasus Press.

# MISCARRIAGE

**Question:** I have been married for a few months and plan on having a baby within the coming year. I've heard the term miscarriage used often, but could you tell me exactly what it means?

**Answer:** Miscarriage is one of those terms that the lay public throws around indiscriminately without necessarily knowing what they are talking about. Miscarriage (also known as spontaneous abortion) is simply the spontaneous interruption of pregnancy up to the 28th week. It is the premature birth of a fetus, so that it does not live. Miscarriage can occur as the result of a bad fall, overactivity or it can just happen without any specific action to provoke the spontaneous interruption. Many physicians view spontaneous abortion as nature's way of rejecting a fetus which has been poorly formed, or had an unhealthy start. They say if spontaneous abortion or miscarriage begins it is best to let it run its course, rather than to try saving a fetus which will be abnormal to full term.

**Question:** Since miscarriage can possibly happen to anyone, without warning, is there any treatment that could be administered at the very start of pregnancy to protect against this happening alogether?

**Answer:** Some physicians have experimented with vitamin E (alpha tocopherol) which was administered to patients from the beginning of pregnancy to the very end. The results have been satisfying as a solid percentage avoided any miscarriage complications, as compared to similar patients who were not administered any vitamin E supplement in controlled dosages. Surely, this lends some support to the idea that alpha tocopherol is helpful in preventing abortion in a large number of cases treated both preventively and therapeutically.

It is further held that the administration of alpha tocopherol just before, or just after conception is helpful in the prevention of congenital defects, and this theory has been borne out in literature concerning animals made vitamin-E deficient by special diets. The

252

placenta is the foundation of good circulation for the fetus. Presumably, if there is a good foundation, a good infant will develop and the mother will remain normal. On the other hand, a defective placenta may alter the whole pregnancy and its product for the worse. The placenta provides the embryo with nutrients of all types, but especially oxygen. Alpha tocopherol has been shown to be an oxygen-conserving agent. This alone would make it a valuable agent in pregnancy. The placenta can also be regarded as a great sponge, a net of capillaries. Their being kept intact is vital to the life of the fetus. Alpha tocopherol has the unique properties of preserving normal capillary strength and in maintaining their proper width. The use of vitamin E in pregnancy is indeed convincing. It is obvious that vitamin E is effective in maintaining the health of the fetus, as well as in providing the fetus with the best possible atmosphere for normal development.

Aside from E, the B vitamins, notably vitamin B1 and niacin, and vitamin C, have shown themselves to be of value in maintaining a normal, comfortable pregnancy. A diet which is rich in foods containing these nutrients, as well as supplementary dosage, is the best guarantee a woman can have for successful pregnancy.

### BIBLIOGRAPHY

Brazelton, T., *Infants and Mothers,* Delacorte Press.

Bronson, Barnard Sawyer, *Nutrition and Food Chemistry,* J. Wiley and Sons, Inc.

Cummings, Richard Osborn, *The American and His Food,* University of Chicago Press.

Davis, Adelle, *Vitality Through Planned Nutrition,* Macmillan Co.

Page, C. E., *How To Feed the Baby to Make It Healthy and Happy,* Health Research Pub.

Rodale, J. I. and Staff, *The Encyclopedia of Common Diseases,* Rodale Books, Inc.

Spotnitz, Hyman and Freeman, Lucy, *How To Be Happy Though Pregnant,* Coward-McCann.

# MULTIPLE SCLEROSIS

**Question:** I know that multiple sclerosis is known as "the crippler" among diseases, but what is the path that this ailment takes in its victim's body?

**Answer:** This disease, which for some reason strikes mainly among young adults, causes the destruction of the protective sheath which covers the nerves of the brain and the spinal cord, acting as an insulation. When this covering is damaged or destroyed and the nerves exposed, the impulses from the brain center cannot pass through them properly, with the result that the muscles which normally do one's bidding are out of control. A progressive weakness ensues. The victim tries to move his leg, but he can't; he tries to focus his eyes, but they remain unfocused; he wills his knees not to buckle, but they do. This is the path of multiple sclerosis, perhaps best illustrated by the brief outline of a typical MS victim's case history.

The patient, apparently well, first felt peculiar pricking sensations in his left foot and leg (pins and needles). Three months later, he complained of a weakness in the knees and blurring vision of the right eye. Soon his balance became poor and he had a tendency to stagger when walking. He felt dizzy upon closing his eyes. In the sixth month, he noticed a continual and severe itching of the face, and with his worsening unsteadiness, it became apparent that he must give up his job. In the ninth month, the patient began to have lapses of memory for recent as well as remote experiences. Finally, he experienced speech difficulties; the fingers of the left hand became numb, and the ordinary motions required for buttoning, tying shoes, etc., became chores that were impossible. The man's vision got worse, but even with glasses he was unable to correct the blurring. He was soon a complete invalid.*

**Question:** Is there a known cause for multiple sclerosis?

**Answer:** The very reason for the occurrence of multiple sclero-

---

*The New York Times,* April 20, 1947, by Howard A. Rusk, M.D.

sis is not known. There have been suggestions that a hereditary influence operates to bring on multiple sclerosis, but the evidence is not very strong. Whenever any genetic influence seems to be present, it is extremely weak and must be reinforced by environmental and constitutional factors. But then, MS (multiple sclerosis) also occurs in persons who have absolutely no history of the disease in the family. From this, it is reasonable to assume that environmental and constitutional factors are the main, and possibly the only, cause of the disease. For some reason, it is known that multiple sclerosis appears most frequently in the colder climates. In the countries of northern Europe the incidence is many times that of countries in the south; in the United States, the incidence of MS in the northern states far outweighs the number of cases in the southern states. Just why cold weather seems to have such an effect no one seems to know.

Experiments have been conducted to indicate a relationship between allergies and MS. It was found that where there is a high percentage of allergic reactions to rye and wheat, in countries where bread is an important food factor, there was a higher percentage of MS cases. Also, there is a low incidence in those countries in which rice is a staple food. Another theory brought forth in medical books is based on a kink in the body's metabolism. Normally, when food is broken down, ammonia is deposited in the nerve cells. This ammonia is quickly removed by other body processes, thus eliminating any chance for poisoning of the nerve cells. In many MS cases, the process for removing the ammonia from the nerve cells failed. It was discovered that a chemical normally present in the body, succinate, when injected into the vein, made possible the removal of ammonia from nerve tissue. This discovery seems to be pertinent, but it is just another theory—still unproven.

**Question:** What of vitamins and diet in relation to multiple sclerosis?

**Answer:** Of all the efforts made at treating multiple sclerosis with a variety of modern drugs and techniques, the use of nutrients and the careful observation of diet have shown the most promising results. One might even say that such measures have shown the only results. There are instances where physicians have used the

B vitamins to achieve some success. The use of thiamin hydro-chloride, given through the spine, to various patients helped some feel, eat, walk and talk. Improvement has been noted in patients treated with niacin (another B vitamin), although the positive condition did not seem to be permanent. A mixture of B6 and hydrocortisone administered through the spine showed some im-provements. The hydrocortisone was used to take advantage of its anti-allergenic and anti-infectious properties, and the vitamin B6 was used for its power to regulate the metabolism of the nerv-ous system.

Another interesting point: because the central nervous system is restricted to the use of glucose for fuel, the level of sugar in the blood is of vital importance, and has direct bearing on the course of any disease in which the spinal cord and the brain are con-cerned. With a diet correcting the sugar level, you are reaching for a healthy system in the body. When one is having trouble with low blood sugar, one notices hunger, fatigue and headache a few hours after eating; and these symptoms disappear immediately after eating. Many persons bring up the blood sugar level with a piece of candy or cake, or a bottle of soda at odd times during the day. But this habit only creates a deeper abyss into which the blood sugar falls when the stimulation of the added sugar wears off. A basis of good nutrition at meal times is what one needs to sustain a steady healthy level of blood sugar.

Of course, all this talk in relation to MS and treatment is still theory, but let us at least realize that there are some things an MS victim can try before giving up his cause as hopeless. Why let a disease take its toll just because no drug company has come up with an antibiotic or a hormone that they claim will arrest the progress of this dread disease? Why not give nature a chance to cure? The treatments with the B vitamins have shown some prom-ise. Why shouldn't a person suffering from multiple sclerosis greatly increase his intake of natural B vitamins, just on the chance that a lack of these could be the root of his troubles? The nerves require the B vitamins for proper function, and MS is a nerve disease. And the correct level of blood sugar is a healthy condition that everyone should strive for, including the MS victim. Good nutrition is of major importance in treating disorders of the nerv-ous system. But good nutrition is important in treating any disease; it is important in simply maintaining good health. Until a multiple sclerosis patient has organized his diet and supplement intake, so that he can feel certain that his body is getting large amounts of all the nutrients it can use, he has not tried everything. He has not tried what could very well be the most important thing of all.

**Question:** I would like to know more about the connection between soil fertilizers and multiple sclerosis.

**Answer:** A good question, as this subject has been brought up in medical journals. It has been noted that the use of inorganic chemicals in farm soils can disturb the mineral balance and natural bacteria of the soil. People whose food comes from soils fertilized with these inorganic fertilizers appear to have more vascular and degenerative diseases than those who use natural organic elements. Of course the connection is obvious: MS is a degenerative disease with vascular involvements. The ruination of our foodstuffs by processing, bleaching and refining, only serves to complete the cycle initiated by inorganic fertilizers to bring to the average person a product that is not rich in the nutritious elements so necessary to good health. And this goes right along with the very basic attitude that improper food is not going to help the victim of multiple sclerosis improve his condition. Since no one is certain just what causes this disease, and we know that a healthy diet helps keep disease away from us on all levels, then the sufferer must be told to put the very best nutriments into his body for maximum functioning capacity.

# MUSCULAR DYSTROPHY

**Question:** What happens to the system of a person who is afflicted with muscular dystrophy?

**Answer:** The disease usually comes on in the form of great muscular weakness in the legs and back, so that the patient has trouble walking. Gradually the paralysis spreads until he is unable to move at all. Respiratory muscles may be affected to such an extent that the patient is unable to cough, so if he contracts even a slight cold, he may suffocate since he cannot cough to remove mucus from his throat or chest. Weakness of legs, lateness in beginning to walk, slowness in running, frequent falls, lordosis (swayback) and prominent stomach—these are easily recognized symptoms of muscular dystrophy in children. In some cases, the disease attacks the arm, shoulder and face muscles before the legs, resulting in a strange expression on the face and possibly inability to close the eyes.

**Question:** Is the disease muscular dystrophy possibly a result of a multiple vitamin deficiency?

**Answer:** We do not know for certain, but there have been a lot of theories related to deficiency of E and B causing some of the symptoms of muscular dystrophy. Experiments with animals (rabbits) have shown that one of the functions of vitamin E in the body is to bring about the synthesis of a substance called acetylcholine from choline (a B vitamin) and acetate. Rabbits who did not have choline in their diet, after a period of time, developed muscular dystrophy. And rabbits, deficient in vitamin E as well, developed muscular dystrophy.

Then by working with a third batch of animals, experimenters gave them large doses of vitamin E, to see to it that the animals were not deficient in vitamin E. And, in this instance, the choline was omitted. Once again, dystrophy symptoms appeared. In this case, they knew for certain that the disease was not produced by an E deficiency, but by a deficiency in choline. In some respects, the kind of disorder produced by choline deficiency is more like that seen in human beings.

With E (a fat-soluble vitamin) we see a closely related functioning to one of the minor B vitamins, as they both pertain to dystrophy. And to add to this theory is also research indicating that the answer may well lie in the body's not being able to use proteins correctly. Perhaps diseases that result in the destruction of vitamin E (such as sprue, celiac disease, and others, involving diarrhea) may also bring about the inability to use proteins properly. Perhaps vitamin E is necessary for proper usage of the protein by the body. But if the relationship exists, the body's deficiencies could bring on this dread disease.

We do not know what causes muscular dystrophy, but all research has pointed to the fact that it is nutritional in origin. Boys are affected more often than girls and the disease quite often afflicts members of the same family. Too, it has been found that the mother often gives a record of very poor diet before the birth of the child who later develops dystrophy. The child may be born after several recurrent abortions, for instance, which appear to indicate serious lack in the diet of many important factors, including vitamin E.

**Question:** Can you give me an idea of the kind of special diet that would be effective in returning a dystrophy victim to health after a diagnosis of "hopeless"?

**Answer:** For one, the diet must be low-cholesterol and low-fat, free of refined sugars and carbohydrates. Only whole grain bread and cereal should be used and make certain it is certified raw milk that the patient is being administered. And lean meat, fish or fowl to supply the correct protein requirements. And nutritional supplements to help the body use the protein correctly. Plenty of vitamin E as well as desiccated liver, which should really be in addition to fresh calves' liver (juice or rare broiled liver) daily. Liver is a wonderful food for all and should particularly be added to a child's diet at the youngest age possible. The fresh raw fruits and vegetables, with extra supplements of vegetable and fruit juices should be eaten daily. Most mothers, these days, try their best to get their children to eat lots of raw fruits and vegetables, but the child who has filled up on candy and ice cream will not necessarily be interested in a raw vegetable. The child with muscular dystrophy symptoms must be made to cut out all "sweets." And finally, lipotropic substances (substances that change fats) such as crude liver and vitamin B12 should be given intramuscularly daily.

## BIBLIOGRAPHY

Albanese, Anthony August, *Protein and Amino Acid Nutrition,* Academic Press.

Bacharach, Alfred Louis, *Science and Nutrition,* Watts and Co.

Bourne, Geoffrey, *Biochemistry and Physiology of Nutrition,* Academic Press.

Bragg, Paul, *Building Powerful Nerve Force,* Health Service, Inc.

Broadstreet, Hobart, *Spine Motion,* The Provoker Press.

Davis, Adelle, *Let's Eat Right to Keep Fit,* Signet Books.

Marsh, A., *How to Be Healthy With Natural Foods,* Arc Books.

Roberts, Sam. E., *Exhaustion—Causes and Treatment,* Rodale Books, Inc.

Rodale, J. I. and Staff, *The Encyclopedia of Common Disease,* Rodale Books, Inc.

Sydenstricker, Edgar, *Health and Environment,* McGraw-Hill.

# INDEX